£25·00
02

D0101928

Tutorial   Registrar

 Barts and The London
Queen Mary's School of Medicine and Dentistry

WHITECHAPEL LIBRARY, TUR   ONDON E1 2AD

Commissioning editor: Melanie Tait
Development editor: Zoë Youd
Production controller: Chris Jarvis
Desk editor: Jackie Holding
Cover designer: Fred Rose

Tutorials for the General Practice Registrar

Edward Warren FRCGP

GP Trainer, Barnsley Vocational Training Scheme;
General Practitioner, Chapelgreen, Sheffield, UK

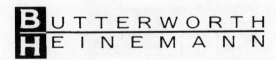

Oxford Auckland Boston Johannesburg Melbourne New Delhi

An imprint of Butterworth-Heinemann
Linacre House, Jordan Hill, Oxford OX2 8DP
225 Wildwood Avenue, Woburn, MA 01801-2041
A division of Reed Educational and Professional Publishing Ltd

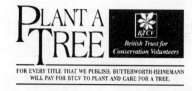 A member of the Reed Elsevier plc group

First published 2002

© Reed Educational and Professional Publishing Ltd 2002

British Library Cataloguing in Publication Data
Warren, Edward
    Tutorials for the general practice registrar
    1.   Family medicine – Great Britain   2.   Physicians (General Practice) –
    Training of – Great Britain
    I.   Title
    362.1'72'071141

Library of Congress Cataloguing in Publication Data
A catalogue reference for this book is available from the Library of Congress

ISBN 0 7506 5322 1

Typeset at Replika Press Pvt Ltd, Delhi 110 040, India
Printed and bound in Great Britain by Martins the Printers,
Berwick-upon-Tweed

For information on all primary care books visit our website at www.bh.com

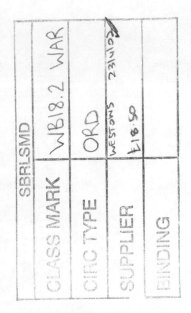

Contents

Acknowledgements

Acknowledgements are due to those people without whom this book would never have been completed. To Melanie Tait at Butterworths who suggested the format for the book and has gently badgered ever since. To Andrew Polmear who reviewed some of the material and left me convinced that he could have made a much better fist of it than I have. To Amar Rughani, partner *extraordinaire*, who jeopardised his marriage by reading the rest of the text until 3 am one morning after I realised that not all the content had been checked for medical accuracy.

And to my wife Dee, and daughters Kate and Jenny who have kept my feet firmly on the ground during the times I was starting to feel important about writing a book. It is sobering indeed when one's literary outpourings have to be adjourned because your 14-year-old daughter wants the computer to email the schoolfriends she has been with all day. Thanks a lot.

Preface

I have recently been visited for re-approval as a trainer. One of the requirements of a GP trainer in my Region is that at least four hours, and preferably five hours a week should be set aside as 'protected teaching time'. In my training days an hour a week was considered the ideal. Learning time set aside from the rush and tumble of day-to-day general practice is still seen as a mark of good training and good learning.

How can such protected time be used to best effect? From an educational point of view, the first call should be time to reflect and consider things that have happened on the job. Being confronted with a genuine dilemma which arises with a real patient in a real surgery focuses the mind wonderfully, whether the mind be that of a GP registrar or a crusty superannuated principal. The bulk of the specified learning time should rightly be taken up with discussion and reflection, by random and problem case analysis, but this does not mean that there is no longer any value in the prepared topic discussion or tutorial.

Even using a curriculum that is appropriately registrar-driven, it is remarkable with what regularity the same tutorial topics are requested by a succession of registrars. The twenty or so chapters in this book are all based on tutorials requested by and discussed with my own registrars. Some have been delivered many times: I have just talked to a registrar about referral to hospital for the fifteenth time in an almost unbroken sequence back to 1993.

To make a tutorial work, trainer and registrar need a shared base of information, and that is what this book tries to provide. A tutorial is not the same thing as a surgery debriefing session, or random or problem case analysis. A tutorial requires that a topic is gone into in some depth, whereas for a debriefing session trainer and registrar have to rely just on the information they happen to be carrying around in their heads at that time. There is nothing wrong in using 'in the head' information, especially as it has usually been committed to memory for a good reason such as recurrent usefulness. On the other hand for a tutorial there is a need to go further.

The material should be read beforehand, and then the tutorial time can be used in its most profitable way: for discussing, clarifying and going off at tangents. All the main facts are supported by reference to the literature, but some may find that the choice of references is a little unorthodox. I make no apology for having used sources which I think most GPs have access to, and hence the liberal use of review articles and cuttings from medical newspapers. They also happen to be the bits of paper which have found their way into my bulging filing cabinet.

Tutorials work best if they are prompted by a particular case the registrar has come across. This means that tutorial topics should be agreed with sufficient notice for preparation to be made, but not so far in advance that the reason for choosing the topic is forgotten. Between one and two weeks is about right. Applying new knowledge to a current problem encourages a deeper level of understanding than the simple recall of that knowledge. Demonstrating how increased knowledge leads to better doctoring is a particularly satisfying tutorial outcome.

The learning objectives offered are simply that – offers. Individual registrars and their trainers will want to add to and subtract from the list depending on circumstances: it is a good idea to discuss the learning objectives at least a day or so before the tutorial so that they can be amended if necessary. Objectives should be SMART: specific, measurable, attainable, relevant, and time-bound.

The text has been set out in the interests of information accessibility rather than literary merit. Boxes and bullet points abound – indeed this preface is probably the longest piece of continuous prose in the whole book. In addition, I have tried to highlight key words and phrases.

A brief summary is added at the end of each topic. If the discussion starts to flag, then I have made some suggestions for issues which it might be worth bringing up. These topics for discussion have largely been chosen because I don't know the answers to them. At the end of the book I have given a list of useful organisations and their websites addresses.

Sitting down for a congenial chat with a like-minded medical colleague is one of the many attractions of being a GP trainer. And they pay you for it as well. Despite all the moaning – and indeed there are plenty of reasons to moan – general practice is still the best job in the world, and training the next generation is a privilege as well as a responsibility. General practice is probably unique in British medical education for providing learners with such close access to an experienced trainer, and long may it continue.

Alcohol abuse

Tutorial aims	**Registrars are aware of the role of alcohol consumption in physical and psychological illness, and are confident in their ability to help alcohol-damaged or at-risk patients.**

Learning objectives

By the end of the tutorial the registrar can:

- List five types of presentation typical in alcohol abuse
- List five dangers of alcohol abuse
- Use a questionnaire to detect alcohol abuse
- Identify the patient physically dependent on alcohol
- List four reasons to refer to a specialist
- Discuss the social role of alcohol
- Discuss the GP's role in alcohol abuse
- Choose appropriate methods to help patients to reduce their alcohol consumption.

A bit of history

The consumption of alcohol has been an important part of social life for thousands of years. Its use is associated with celebrations and good times, with sociability and comradeship. The first recorded brewing was in 5000 BC when beer was part of the daily wages of the temple workers in Mesopotamia. William Pitt the Younger is alleged to have drunk 574 bottles of claret, 854 of Madeira, and 2410 of port in a single year.

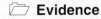 **Evidence**

Historic use of alcohol

- Total consumption lowest in 1940: consumption same in 1980 as in 1900[1]
- Use of spirits falling, and wine rising
- In 1700, beer consumption per head was about 10 times what it was in 1980[1]
- Recent increased consumption mostly in women and in the 18 to 25 year age group[2]
- The cost of alcohol halved relative to average wages between 1950 and 1980.[3]

The 'unit' of alcohol

Alcohol consumption is measured in 'units', and alcohol-related dangers are commonly discussed in relation to these units. One unit contains between 8 g and 10 g of pure alcohol. For convenience it is assumed that this amount is contained in half a pint of ordinary strength beer or lager, one glass of wine or a 'pub' measure of spirits. Home measures are generally about twice pub measures.

The unit of alcohol is clearly an imprecise measure. Some beers have twice the alcohol content of others. Wines can vary in strength from 5% to 13% alcohol. A 750 ml bottle of 40% strength whisky contains 300 g of alcohol: thirty 10 g units or nearly forty 8 g units. In assessing the risks of excess consumption, no account is taken of body weight.

How much do people drink?

Most adults in the United Kingdom drink some alcohol. One in eight 13-year-olds and half of 15-year-olds are drinking alcohol at least once a week.[4]

📁 Evidence

Adult alcohol consumption per week[5]

	Men		Women
Nil	6%		11%
Under 5 units	38%		65%
5–20 units	30%		20%
20–35 units	13%		2%
35–50 units	8%	Over 35 units	2%
Over 50 units	6%		

'Safe' drinking

All-cause *mortality* is lowest for men who drink between 7 and 21 units of alcohol a week[6] and for women who drink under 14 units a week.[7] Most alcohol risks are dose-related, but abstinence is associated with an increased risk of coronary heart disease (CHD),[6] and since CHD is such an important cause of death the figures are distorted. The British medical establishment supports upper *limits* of 21 units for men and 14 units for women, and suggests that drinking 'for the good of your heart' is not sensible. The British government previously had the same policy, but in 1995 an interdepartmental working group, composed entirely of civil servants, changed their 'sensible drinking' limits to 21 units for women and 28 units for men. They did however make the important point that *binge drinking* is dangerous even if the overall weekly limit is adhered to.[8]

Drinkers can be divided into four categories

- *Social drinkers*: those who keep to the limits are unlikely to become damaged
- *At-risk drinkers*: drinking over the limit, a potential risk to health
- *Problem drinkers*: damage is occurring
- *Physically dependent/addicted*.

In an average GP list of 2000, there will be

- about seven physically dependent drinkers[3] (of whom half will be known)[9]
- up to 40 problem drinkers (of whom a fifth will be known).[3]

Up to 12% of men and 2% of women over 65 are problem drinkers.[10] The problems caused are made worse by frailty, coexisting illnesses and medication. Some occupational groups, for instance publicans and doctors, drink more than average amounts of alcohol.[1]

The dangers of alcohol overuse

Only about one in ten adults in Britain do not drink alcohol at all. The minority of men who drink over 50 units a week and women who drink over 36 units a week are at clear risk of damage. The risks of alcohol damage rise with the level of consumption, but accurately predicting the effect of excessive drinking in an individual patient is most difficult. Some people appear undamaged after a lifetime of heavy drinking, while others are damaged at much lower levels of consumption. From the GP perspective, an 'at-risk' drinker is drinking over the recommended limits but as yet there is no obvious harm done (and there may never be). On the other hand, the 'problem' drinker is already experiencing damage, whatever their actual consumption is.

Very heavy drinkers suffer the most damage, but they are few in number. There are many more people in the 'at-risk' and 'problem' categories, and the cumulative damage in this group exceeds that in the 'dependent' group. This is also the group with which a GP is likely to have most contact, and may be able to help.

1. Death
There are estimated to be 28 000 excess deaths per year in the UK because of alcohol.[11]

2. Heart disease
The increase in heart disease seen in heavy drinkers does not become apparent until consumption levels are over 40 unit a week.[12]

Some types of alcoholic drink may be safer than others. This might explain the *French paradox*: although alcohol consumption in France is high by international standards, nonetheless the heart attack rate is low. From this it is speculated that red wine in particular may have protective properties. Red wine contains many things as well as alcohol, and it may be the anti-oxidants and trace elements which have a beneficial effect on blood coagulability.[13] Regular (as opposed to binge) drinking seems more beneficial, as does drinking with meals.[14]

3. Hypertension
In up to 30% of cases of hypertension, alcohol is the principal or sole cause. This effect is reversible on abstinence.[15] Accordingly the risk of stroke rises with alcohol consumption.

4. Cancer
Alcohol is implicated in 3% of all cancer deaths, around 4300 a year. Cancers

of the mouth, pharynx, larynx, liver and oesophagus are definitely, and of breast and rectum probably, related to alcohol consumption.[16]

5. Road accidents

Alcohol is responsible for about 1000 road traffic accident (RTA) deaths per year, or 20% of the total. Up to 50% of persons killed in RTAs are over the legal alcohol driving limit. Between 10 pm and 4 am on Friday and Saturday nights, two thirds of drivers and motorbike riders have alcohol levels above the *legal limit*. Drinking is involved in 45% of road accidents with young people.[17]

6. Other accidents

Alcohol is involved in 50% of murders, 20% of cases of child abuse, 65% of suicides, 20% of drownings, 35% of domestic accidents and 60% of serious head injuries.[18]

A fifth of people admitted to hospitals have problems with alcohol abuse.[5] Overall, 14% of attendances at accident and emergency departments are due to alcohol, but between 8 pm and midnight the figure is 24%, and from midnight to 6 am it is 46%.[9]

7. Drinking and pregnancy[2]

The risk of spontaneous *abortion* is increased in women who drink alcohol when pregnant. The *Fetal Alcohol Syndrome* affects 1 to 2 of 1000 live births, and may be seen when the mother has drunk more than 70 units a week during pregnancy. *Fetal Alcohol Effects* are seen in 2 to 3 of 1000 live births, and may be brought about by maternal drinking over 35 units a week during pregnancy. Up to 8% of all mental retardation may be attributable to alcohol ingestion. A pregnant woman who drinks 10 units a week approximately doubles the risk of a small-for-dates baby. There is probably no completely safe level of drinking during pregnancy, but failing complete abstinence it is advisable to limit intake to two units on any given occasion.

The economics of alcohol

The overall cost of alcohol excess in the UK was estimated in 1985 at £2 billion[19] (over £5 billion in 2001 prices), and the cost of alcohol abuse to the NHS is estimated to be £3 billion a year.[20]

The alcoholic drinks market is worth (1999) £25 billion a year (of which a sizeable chunk goes to the government as duty) and employs a million people. There is one public house for every 550 adults, or between 2 and 3 per GP.[21]

Intervening in alcohol abuse

Two strategies have been proposed for reducing alcohol damage:

- *High-risk approach.* The small group of heavy drinkers are targeted for treatment
- *Population approach.* The aim is to reduce the average alcohol consumption in the general population. The majority of alcohol damage is seen in the

large numbers of people who drink only slightly more than is good for them.

In fact the two approaches are not conflicting. The number of alcohol-damaged people in a community is closely related to the average alcohol consumption of that community. A general reduction in consumption will hence reduce the numbers of problem drinkers. The heavier drinkers reduce their consumption as well as the lighter drinkers.[22]

The Department of Health estimates that a 1% increase in the *price* of alcohol leads to a 1% reduction in consumption.[11] However, alcohol is big business with significant revenue implications. This may explain the lukewarm attitude of successive governments towards controlling alcohol consumption through fiscal means.

Assessing alcohol consumption

Ask

People are becoming more accustomed to enquiries about aspects of their lifestyle, including alcohol use. Details are needed by insurance companies, and the GP contract requires a record of admitted alcohol consumption. Asking about alcohol is unlikely to cause offence. If there is reluctance to disclose drinking behaviour, this may in itself help with a diagnosis. If alcohol may be contributing to a problem, it is appropriate to explain that all possible causes of the illness should be explored.

People may not admit how much they drink

- There may be guilt about the drinking
- Genuine errors may be made in estimating the amount drunk
- Patients may not wish their symptoms to be dismissed as due to alcohol for fear of a more serious pathology being missed.

The 'Drink Diary'

If a drinking problem is suspected, a drinking history can be taken by reference to the last seven days. Many problem drinkers will tell you that the last week has been unusual in some respect leading to more than average consumption.[5] The history can be reinforced by inviting the patient to fill in a Drink Diary. A number of published examples are available.[23] On each day record:

- How much was drunk
- What were the circumstances of the drinking
- Feelings before and after the drinking
- What if any were the consequences of the drinking.

Over the course of a week or two it will be possible to get an accurate assessment of the amount drunk, and also get some insight into why the drinking behaviour is occurring.

Recognising a problem drinker

Suspicious presentations

Some clinical presentations should make the GP suspect that alcohol consumption is causing damage.

📄 **Guidelines**   **Presentations indicating possible alcohol damage[5]**

Physical

- Gastro-intestinal symptoms e.g. vomiting, diarrhoea, '*Monday morning gastritis*'
- Hypertension
- Jaundice
- Collapse, fits, faints
- Fractures, especially rib fractures
- Trauma e.g. injuries, accidents, burns
- Withdrawal symptoms: shakes, night sweats
- Presenting at the surgery smelling of alcohol
- Obesity, especially in young males.

Psychological

- Anxiety symptoms
- Sexual problems
- Inappropriate behaviour in surgery
- Depression
- Drug abuse, especially benzodiazepines.

Familial

- Spouse battering
- Child abuse
- Psychological problems in spouse
- Psychological problems in children.

Social

- Financial problems, debt
- Legal problems, criminal, civil, driving offences
- Work problems, absenteeism, frequent job change, dismissal.

Five-shot Questionnaire[24]

The use of questionnaires is known to increase the GP detection rate of problem drinkers.[11] On average, GPs know of only a third of those patients who are abusing alcohol. The use of the five-shot questionnaire will detect about twice this number: at a cut-off of < 2.5, it has a sensitivity of 74% and a specificity of 81% for alcohol abuse or dependence.[24] However two out of three patients who test positive on this questionnaire do not have an alcohol problem (positive predictive value 36% for women, 38% for men)[24] and so a positive result should prompt further investigation.

📄 **Guidelines**   **The five-shot questionnaire[25]**

1. How often do you have a drink containing alcohol?
never	(0.0)
monthly or less	(0.5)
two to four times a month	(1.0)
two to three times a week	(1.5)
four or more times a week	(2.0)

2. How many drinks containing alcohol do you have on a typical day when you are drinking?
one or two	(0.0)
three or four	(0.5)
five or six	(1.0)
seven to nine	(1.5)
ten or more	(2.0)

3. Have people ever annoyed you by criticising your drinking?
no	(0.0)
yes	(1.0)

4. Have you ever felt bad or guilty about your drinking?
no	(0.0)
yes	(1.0)

5. Have you ever had a drink first thing in the morning to steady your nerves or to get rid of a hangover?
no	(0.0)
yes	(1.0)

The 'at-risk' drinker

Some people will show no signs of alcohol damage, but will be drinking at a level which may cause problems in the future. This group should be encouraged to reduce their drinking to a safe level. General advice or even a leaflet may help. A number of people find they are drinking more than they mean to, and the following tips will help to prevent this.

📄 **Guidelines**   **Tips to reduce alcohol use[5]**

- Occupy yourself e.g. play a game, or talk, or eat
- Change the drink (breaks old habits)
- Imitate the slow drinker
- Put the glass down between sips
- Try to avoid rounds, or miss yourself out on your round
- Eat first (the alcohol absorption is slowed)
- Take days off drinking altogether
- Learn to refuse drinks (this may take practice)
- Take smaller sips
- Drink for the taste
- Dilute spirits
- Start later

The physically dependent drinker

Patients who get alcohol withdrawal symptoms are physically dependent, and are best dealt with by psychiatrists. The chance of a withdrawal syndrome is greatest with heavier drinkers, but the amount consumed is not the only consideration when assessing the likelihood of a withdrawal reaction.[26]

- Withdrawal symptoms begin after three to six hours without drinking, and last five to seven days, or occasionally longer
- Up to 12 hours the early symptoms are of tremor, sweating, anorexia, nausea, insomnia and anxiety
- Between 10 and 60 hours there is a risk of withdrawal seizures. These are generalised and may precede or accompany delirium tremens
- After 72 hours delirium tremens may occur, with severe tremor, confusion, disorientation, agitation, visual and auditory hallucinations and paranoid ideation. Around 5% of patients withdrawing from alcohol in hospital develop delirium tremens, and 10% of these die.[23]

Most patients needing detoxification will require admission to hospital, sometimes under the medical team and sometimes under the psychiatrists, depending on the local arrangement.

🗎 Guidelines

Detoxification may be possible at home if[27]

- Patient physically healthy
- Good family support
- No past withdrawal seizures or delirium tremens
- No recent failed home detoxification
- No suicidal risk or polysubstance abuse.

Withdrawal symptoms can be relieved using a benzodiazepine, usually chlordiazepoxide at a dose of 10 to 15 mg three or four times a day, with a maximum of 40 mg four times a day. The dose is tailed off to zero over seven to ten days. Chlormethiazole is now only considered safe for hospital practice because of the risk of dependency and of respiratory depression.[26]

The GP's role in helping alcohol-damaged patients

GPs are in an ideal position to help patients with alcohol problems. They have contact with a majority of patients each year, contacts are usually patient-initiated so that someone who presents with an alcohol problem has presumably decided that a problem exists.[28] 'Brief intervention' has been shown to reduce alcohol consumption by an average of a fifth in heavy drinkers.[11] Brief intervention consists of

- An assessment of alcohol intake
- Provision of information on hazardous or harmful drinking
- Clear advice to cut down or stop drinking.

Most GP think they ought to do more for problem drinkers, but under half actually do so,[28] being concerned about time constraints, lack of skills and the possibility of opening a 'can of worms'.

The presence of alcohol damage usually comes to light in one of four ways, in order of frequency.

- A physical or emotional crisis has arisen because of drinking. Four fifths of patients referred for treatment of alcohol misuse have important medical problems[3]
- A spouse or other family member or a friend attends to tell of their suspicions
- A patient presents with a problem which may be related to drinking
- Evidence of alcohol damage and excess consumption is detected during routine screening.

It is important to take notice of what concerned *carers* may say, as their assessment will often be more accurate than the story obtained from the patient. In addition, it is the carers that have to put up with the results of the drinking, and so they deserve consideration. Carers are also a crucial part of attempts at treatment.

This said, treatment cannot be imposed. Patients must be sufficiently aware that their drinking is causing or at least aggravating a problem to present for help. Such awareness may not be permanent, so that one day they will admit the drink is a problem, and the next they may be equally convinced that the only reason they drink is because the world is so awful.

A *psychiatric illness* will commonly co-exist with the heavy drinking, and it is often difficult to sort out whether the psychiatric problem or the drink problem is the primary cause of the symptoms. Patients tend to underestimate the relative effect of drinking. Whatever psychological disorder may be present, the overuse of alcohol will certainly make things worse, and things are unlikely to improve unless the drinking is reduced.

Making the change

Many heavy drinkers do not think they have a problem. According to the *Stages of Change* model[29] they are at the 'pre-contemplation' stage of awareness. To them there is no reason to see a doctor or anyone else about their drinking, and their existence may only come to medical attention because of the concern of relatives. Others may have begun to think about their drinking but are not convinced that reduction will do any good. They are at the *'contemplation'* stage. It may be possible to nudge these patients through into the next stage where they are ready to take action about their drinking, the *'preparation'* stage, and then into the *'action'* stage of awareness when reduction of consumption can be achieved.

Motivational Interviewing[30] is a technique designed to move a patient along to the next stage of awareness, and is based on two observations:

- If you express a viewpoint, then your patient will tend to take the opposite view
- If people say something often enough, they will come to believe it.

It follows that hounding a patient to reduce their drinking will be counter-productive.

- Work within the patient's own framework. It is not only people who think of themselves as 'alcoholic' who may want to cut down. And don't make assumptions: a desire to cut down may be the result of worry about cost or weight gain, rather than worry over health and the marriage

- Discuss the advantages and disadvantages of drinking and not drinking. Such a *'profit and loss balance'* should include mainly the reasons the patient gives, but the GP may offer suggestions
- In discussion, pick out statements which demonstrate the *patient's own reasons* for cutting down
- Encourage patients to emphasise their own role in the drinking behaviour. They can always choose to drink less, and it's no good constantly blaming external factors
- Sympathise with the wish to alter drinking habits, and also with the difficulty of doing so
- Use facts rather than opinions. There will be the drinking history or drinking diary. Patients can be told how their alcohol consumption compares with others. Blood tests can be used as a stimulus for change, and also as an ongoing record of progress. Mean corpuscular volume (MCV) is raised in about 50% of alcohol dependent patients (compared with up to 2% of the general population). A raised gamma glutamyl transferase (GGT) and MCV will identify 90% of the alcohol dependent.[7] However, blood tests are not as good as questionnaires for detecting alcohol abuse[24]
- Use *cognitive dissonance*: this is a technique using patients' own expressed feelings to encourage reduced consumption, e.g. 'You say that you drink because you are always broke, but then your drinking is costing you £100 a week'; 'You say you drink because your wife doesn't love you, but then she only shouts at you when you get home drunk. I don't understand'.

Staying stopped

Progress should be reviewed at intervals. Success should be praised and a further attempt encouraged if there has been a lapse. Motivation to stop may not always be present. It often takes several goes before success.

- Look for what has triggered any relapse. Avoiding the trigger may help future attempts
- Keep contact with other family members and any other health workers who have been involved. It is best if everybody concerned is saying the same things. A united front is required
- Continue to monitor input, and reinforce with repeated blood tests if needed. Enquire about other problems e.g. impotence, work problems.

Cravings

As alcohol is a tranquilliser, its withdrawal may be associated with anxiety symptoms. Anxiety and the fear of anxiety may be equally troublesome. Anxiety-lowering techniques may help, such as sequential muscle contraction or breathing exercises. More complex devices such as meditation or relaxation tapes may be useful.

Resources

The above package of brief intervention takes about 10 to 15 minutes on up to four occasions.[11] This is rather more than standard care, but then the stakes are quite high.

Problem situations

1. **Suicide threats**. The suicide rate is high in alcohol abusers, and drunkenness may lower the threshold for an impetuous act. An assessment must be made of suicide risk, and if this is significant then admission may be needed. The Mental Health Act can be used if the patient is at risk of self-harm.
2. **Violence**. This is common, and the police may need to be involved. Consider child abuse procedures if appropriate. Delusional jealousy among husbands is particularly troublesome.
3. **Drunk in the surgery**. Once may be tolerated, but it is impossible to do useful work with someone who is drunk.

Reasons to refer

Some alcohol-damaged patients will need inpatient care because

- De-toxification is needed
- Treatment for an alcohol-induced illness is needed
- Psychological symptoms are so severe that patients are a danger to themselves or others.

A patient who is not acutely unwell may still benefit from a planned admission to withdraw from the alcohol.

Outpatient referral will be appropriate for those who

- Are not responding to community treatment
- Have complicating co-existing psychiatric or physical problems.

Where a physical illness is causing concern it will be necessary to take advice from the medical team rather than the psychiatrists.

Other members of the primary health care team can be involved. The key workers here are the *community psychiatric nurses*. In some areas there may be a *community alcohol team* who can be referred to. In addition, most alcohol-dependent patients would benefit from contact with one of the self-help organisations involved in alcohol work.

📄 Guidelines

Reasons to refer

- No progress with treatment
- Serious medical complications, e.g. cirrhosis
- Severe withdrawal symptoms especially if there have been fits or delirium tremens
- Home support is poor
- Complicating psychological or family factors
- Treatment with disulfiram or acamprosate is being considered. Use of these drugs should be restricted to problem cases under specialist care.

Self-help groups

1. *Alcoholics Anonymous* is a voluntary fellowship of the alcohol-dependent who help each other through group meetings and a *12-step programme* to recovery. There are about 2300 groups around the country. Some people are unable to tolerate the slightly religious attitude to the problem. The address is:

> Alcoholics Anonymous,
> PO Box 1,
> Stonebow House,
> Stonebow,
> York YO1 2NJ.
> Tel: (01904) 644026.
> www.alcoholics-anonymous.org

2. *Al-Anon* is a self-help group for the family and friends of problem drinkers. There are over 1000 local groups. *Alateen* is a subsection for teenagers whose lives are being affected by somebody else's drinking. The address is:

> Al-Anon,
> 61, Great Dover Street,
> London SE1 4YF
> Tel 020 7430 0888.
> www.hexnet.co.uk/alanon

3. *Councils on Alcoholism* is a voluntary organisation where counselling is offered to drinkers and families. Councils exist in most biggish population centres.

Summary

- Each year in the UK alcohol kills 28 000 people, the second biggest mortality (i.e. after tobacco) of any drug
- Only a small minority of the alcohol-damaged are dependent/addicted drinkers
- GP intervention has a small but worthwhile effect, and is not too time-consuming
- Most alcohol abusers will need several attempts before reducing consumption
- Alcohol abusers are more likely to be influenced by their own reasons for stopping than they are by reasons imposed by others
- Alcohol-dependent patients, and those in whom primary care management has failed, need specialist referral.

Topics for discussion

- A 1% increase in the duty on alcohol results in a 1% reduction in consumption.[10] The government should reduce alcohol consumption by increasing alcohol duty
- It's a good man who can hold his drink
- The sponsorship of sport by the alcohol industry should be banned
- Licensing laws should be abandoned as they are unworkable and have little effect

- Health workers should set a good example by abstinence from alcohol
- You can't trust an alcoholic.

📖 **References**

1. RCGP. Report from General Practice No. 24. *Alcohol – a balanced view.* London, 1986.
2. BMA symposium, 30th November 1983. *Alcohol and child development.* London, 1983.
3. Ashworth M and Gerada C. ABC of mental health. Addiction and dependence. Part II: Alcohol. *BMJ*, 1997; 315: 358–60.
4. Hoskins T. Alcohol abuse in children. *Mat Child Health* 1988; 14: 194–6.
5. Medical Council on Alcoholism. *Hazardous Drinking.*1987: London.
6. Doll R, Peto R, Hall E et al. Mortality in relation to consumption of alcohol: 13 years' observation on male British doctors. *BMJ* 1994; 309: 911–8.
7. Bloor R N. Social Drinker? Detecting and assessing alcohol problems. *Update* 1993; 47: 24–30.
8. Edwards G. Sensible drinking. *BMJ* 1996; 312: 1.
9. Anderson P. Alcohol epidemiology. *Practitioner* 1991; 235: 594.
10. Dunne F J. Misuse of alcohol or drugs by elderly people. *BMJ* 1994; 308: 608–9.
11. CRD. Brief interventions and alcohol use, *Effective Health Care* 1993; 1(7); The Royal Society of Medicine Press Ltd. Nuffield Institute for Health, University of Leeds; Centre for Health Economics, University of York; Research Unit, Royal College of Physicians.
12. Kemm J. Alcohol and heart disease: the implications of the U-shaped curve. *BMJ* 1993; 307: 1373–4.
13. British Heart Foundation. *Alcohol and cardiovascular diseases.* 1993; Factfile 10/93.
14. British Heart Foundation. *Alcohol and cardiovascular disease.* 1998; Factfile 1/98.
15. Sanders J B. Alcohol: an important cause of hypertension. *BMJ* 1987; 294: 1045–6.
16. Austoker J. Reducing alcohol intake. *BMJ* 1994; 308: 1549–52.
17. Thomson A D (ed). *Licence to kill?* Alcoholism No 3. 1987; Medical council on alcoholism.
18. The Guardian, 23rd May, 1992.
19. Wallace P. Effectiveness of alcohol intervention. *Update* 1995; 51: 834–7.
20. *BMA News*, 2 June 2001.
21. Abraham T. Primary care needs to address alcohol consumption nationally. *General Practitioner* 1999; 8 January.
22. Dillner L. Alcohol abuse. *BMJ* 1991; 02: 859–60.
23. Health Education Authority/Alcohol Concern. *Rx cut down on your drinking*, 1987; London.
24. Aertgeerts B, Buntinx F, Ansoms S et al. Screening properties of questionnaires and laboratory tests for the detection of alcohol abuse or dependence in a general practice population. *Br J Gen Pract* 2001; 51: 206–17.
25. Aertgeerts B and Buntinx F. Screening for alcohol abuse. (Letter). *Br J Gen Pract* 2001; 51: 492–3.
26. Drug and Therapeutic. Alcohol problems in the general hospital. *Drug Ther Bull* 1991; 29: 69–71.
27. Drug and Therapeutic. Managing the heavy drinker in primary care. *Drug Ther Bull* 2000; 38(8): 60–4.

28. Deehan A, Marshall E J and Strang J. Tackling alcohol misuse: opportunities and obstacles in primary care. *Br J Gen Pract* 1998; 48: 1779–82.
29. Johnstone C. Effective brief intervention in problem drinking. *Practitioner* 1999; 243: 614–18.
30. Miller W R. Motivational interviewing with problem drinkers. *Behavioural Psychotherapy* 1983; 11: 147–72.

Anxiety management in primary care

Tutorial aim	**The registrar can manage most cases of anxiety in general practice.**
Learning objectives	By the end of the tutorial the registrar can:

- List five symptoms of anxiety
- Describe four types of anxiety
- Discuss the stigma attached to the diagnosis anxiety
- List five differential diagnoses of anxiety
- Discuss the role of medication in treatment of anxiety
- Help an anxious patient choose the best treatment.

Introduction

- At any one time between 3 and 5% of the adult population suffer generalised anxiety disorder or panic disorder, women being slightly more commonly affected than men[1]
- In any six-month period, 10% of the population will suffer an anxiety disorder[2]
- In a given year 65% of people will experience lesser degrees of anxiety or emotional disorder.[3]

Under half of patients who suffer anxiety will consult their GP about it,[2] but such are the numbers involved that each GP will each year conduct 180 consultations with patients for anxiety.[3] At least 15% of patients attending GP surgeries will have some symptoms of anxiety.[1] As will be discussed later, patients with some types of anxiety are more likely to consult than others.[2]

- Anxiety states account for about 20% of hospital psychiatric admissions, and 40% of psychiatric outpatient consultations[4]
- The UK cost of anxiety was estimated in 1994 at £5.6 billion a year (£7.5 billion at 2001 prices), equivalent to a third of all NHS expenditure at the time.[5]

Stress or anxiety?

All people experience stress from their environment. A certain amount of stress has a motivating effect, and the consequent achievement improves self-esteem. At this level, stress improves well-being.

As environmental stress increases, so does performance, but only up to a point. Beyond this threshold, people begin to feel less well, and function less efficiently. Eventually this can lead to a catastrophic loss of emotional well-being and productivity, as is seen in *burnout*. The ability to withstand stress varies between people, and varies in the same person at different times. A stress coped with by one person may be intolerable to another. The effects of stress are cumulative, so that an extra seemingly minor worry may tip the balance into illness.

The symptoms of stress and anxiety are the same. Patients with anxiety are often being made worse by stresses in their environment. The difference between anxiety and stress is that in anxiety the symptoms experienced are more severe than might be expected from the circumstances, whereas in stress the symptoms are appropriate to the circumstances.

The diagnosis 'anxiety' carries *stigma* for many sufferers. It is seen as a weakness or a lack of courage or of moral fibre. Stress on the other hand is a legitimate response to circumstances, and is associated with higher-status occupations. The current wealth of literature on the emotional problems of GPs refers to stress rather than anxiety disorder, so even doctors are not immune from the stigma.

The judgement about whether the levels of stress are sufficient to explain or justify the patient's symptoms can be a difficult one. GPs as a group are pretty good at withstanding stress, or at least imagine themselves to be, and so may not be very good at understanding the impact of the stress being experienced by others. It is a person's *perceived level* of stress which is important.

In practical terms it does not much matter whether the problem is stress or anxiety. A management plan for either stress or anxiety must take account of the circumstances in which it occurs. Reducing as far as possible the stress (or perceived stress) of the environment is an important aim of treatment. By using the term 'stress' the patient can maintain self-esteem, an important part of any anxiety management plan. The only disadvantage of maintaining this slight deceit is that the stigma of anxiety remains unchallenged.

Scoring systems have been devised to help quantify the amount of stress being experienced by a person. Highlights from one such system show that the death of a partner is twice as stressful as getting married, about four times as stressful as having trouble with the 'in-laws' and eight times as stressful as the approach of Christmas. The occurrence of stressful events may nearly double the risk of a major illness (either physical or emotional) in the subsequent two years.[6]

Diagnosing anxiety

The symptoms of anxiety are shown in the box. The differential diagnosis of anxiety is not extensive, unless it is associated with a lot of autonomic symptoms. Physical disorders which may mimic anxiety include:

- Thyrotoxicosis
- Phaeochromocytoma
- Consumption of alcohol and other drugs should be enquired after. Four or more cups of coffee or tea a day, or the equivalent in other caffeine-containing drinks are enough to produce symptoms of anxiety[7]
- When a lot of autonomic symptoms are present, the differential diagnosis widens hugely to include most cardiac, respiratory and neurological disorders.

If there is doubt about the diagnosis, further help can be obtained using a questionnaire. The one in the box derives from the work of Goldberg in Manchester. The most important psychological illness which may present with symptoms similar to anxiety is depression. In addition, *depression and anxiety often co-exist*. The presence of the typical symptoms of depression will confirm the diagnosis. If depression is present with anxiety, treating the depression will often improve the anxiety.[8]

📄 Guidelines   Symptoms of anxiety[8]

- Inner tension
- A feeling of impending doom
- Worrying about trifles
- Difficulty falling asleep
- Loss of appetite (however, some sufferers eat more)
- Difficulty concentrating due to distractibility
- Agitation
- Autonomic symptoms[4]

   palpitations
   sweating
   dyspepsia or diarrhoea
   urinary frequency or urgency
   dry mouth
   blurred vision
   tremor.

📄 Guidelines   Questionnaire to diagnose anxiety[9]

Score one for each 'yes':

1. Have you felt keyed up, on edge?
2. Have you been worrying a lot?
3. Have you been irritable?
4. Have you had difficulty relaxing?

If 'yes' to three or more questions, go on to:

5. Have you been sleeping poorly?
6. Have you had headaches or neck ache?
7. Have you had any of the following: trembling, tingling, dizzy spells, sweating, urinary frequency, diarrhoea?

8. Have you been worried about your health?
9. Have you had difficulty falling asleep?

A total score of 6 or more predicts a 50% chance of a clinically important anxiety disorder.

The anxiety disorders

The term 'anxiety' covers a number of different diagnoses. Different treatments are of different value in the different disorders.

Generalised anxiety disorder (GAD)

This is probably a group of conditions rather than a single condition. All are characterised by anxiety accompanied by mild depressive features. Symptoms include:[10]

- No clear object of concern
- Trembling, restlessness, autonomic overactivity
- Trouble getting to sleep
- Wide range of situations interpreted as threatening
- Commonly associated with depression.

About 4% of a typical GP list will have GAD, and about a quarter of them will have *consulted* their GP.[2] *Cognitive therapy*, for at least six months, does better than diazepam or placebo in the treatment of GAD.[11] In addition, it can be combined effectively into a broader package of anxiety management.

Panic disorder

Characteristics of panic disorder are:[2]

- Episodes of panic, including *physical symptoms* such as dyspnoea, dizziness, palpitations, trembling, sweating and fear of dying
- It can occur with agoraphobia or social phobia
- Commonly associated with *depression*
- The episodes of panic are not related to a phobic stimulus, and so are in that sense *inexplicable*[8]
- The illness is *maintained by fear of the immediate consequences* of an attack and the significance of any accompanying physical symptoms.[12]

Around 1% of the population suffer from panic disorder, and half of them will consult.[2]

The tricyclic antidepressant *imipramine* is effective in panic disorder.[13] Full benefit is obtained with normal antidepressant doses (75 to 200 mg a day) and may take several weeks to achieve. The starting dose should be small. Similar efficacy has been shown for monoamine oxidase inhibitors, particularly *phenelzine*, but the use of such medication has fallen from favour because of concerns over interactions with some foods.

High-dose *benzodiazepines* work in panic disorder.[14] However, benefit requires long-term use, with all its attendant dangers. Also, benzodiazepine *withdrawal symptoms* are very similar to a panic attack, and so when withdrawing treatment it is difficult to say whether symptoms are due to the re-emergence of the panic disorder, or to benzodiazepine withdrawal.[13] Following advice from the Committee on the Safety of Medicines (CSM), the data sheets for benzodiazepines have been amended so that they are only indicated for short-term use in anxiety.[15]

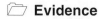 **Evidence**

> **The treatment of panic disorder[16]**
>
> - 87% of patients improve after 15 weekly sessions of Cognitive Therapy
> - 50% improve on benzodiazepine
> - 36% improve on placebo.

Phobic Disorders

Social phobia is the anxiety which some people feel when in social situations such as at a party, or eating out in a restaurant. *Agoraphobia* is the anxiety experienced by some people when they are away from home, or in a crowded place where it is difficult to leave. The anxiety may induce episodes of panic. Other *simple phobias*, such as problems with spiders, are generally less disabling.

Phobic patients will tend to avoid circumstances which have caused them problems in the past. The anxiety caused by *avoiding phobic situations* adds to the symptoms. The fear of the situation becomes worse than the situation itself. Up to 10% of adults have some phobic symptoms, but only about a tenth of these consult a doctor because of them.[2] The patients who do consult will on average have had their symptoms for nine years.[17]

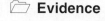 **Evidence**

> **Treating phobias[18]**
>
> In phobic conditions
>
> - *Graded exposure* will bring about lasting improvement in 60%
> - Only 25% secure complete recovery
> - Teaching of anxiety management probably improves the outcome.

Obsessive compulsive disorder

Obsessive compulsive disorder is characterised by

- Obsessional thoughts or compulsive actions. Common forms are incessant hand washing or checking
- The patient is fully aware that their obsessive thoughts and activities are senseless. On the other hand not doing the action leads to high levels of anxiety.

About 1% of adults suffer obsessive compulsive disorder, but only a fifth of these will consult a doctor.[2]

Post-traumatic stress disorder

This is a reaction to a very stressful event, either physical or emotional. *Within six months of the event* there is

- Persistent remembering or reliving of the stress by intrusive *flashbacks*, vivid memories or recurring *dreams*
- Distress when exposed to (or avoiding) circumstances associated with the *trigger stress*
- Psychogenic *amnesia* or persistently increased psychological *sensitivity* and arousal plus *at least two* of:

> difficulty falling or staying asleep
> irritability
> difficulty concentrating
> distractibility
> increased restlessness
> apprehension.

Treatment by supportive *counselling* is usually worth a try, but the long-term *outlook for the patient is uncertain.*[19]

Acute anxiety

Anxiety can come on very quickly, especially in people who have a background of problems. Most presentations of acute anxiety are in patients *already known* to the GP or psychiatric services. The autonomic symptoms may be so severe that an imminent heart attack or stroke is feared: such fears are fuelled by the anxiety. Casualty departments probably see more of such cases than do GPs. Symptoms include palpitations, breathlessness, chest pains and tingling in the lips and extremities: all symptoms which are found in serious physical illness. The sufferer will be restless, agitated and wide-eyed.

Hyperventilation may be found in association with acute anxiety. Overbreathing reduces blood levels of carbon dioxide, causing alkalosis. This brings about spontaneous discharge of the peripheral nerves, which manifests itself as tetany and paraesthesiae in the motor and sensory nerves respectively. The tetany leads to breathlessness and a crushing chest pain, and the sensory involvement causes the 'pins and needles' sensation.

There may have been a recent severe shock or a family argument which has generated anxiety.

Apart from the agitation and the sense of urgency which the patient imparts, and probably a tachycardia, there may be little else to find on clinical examination. In a calm and unhurried manner, it is appropriate to check the pulse and listen to the heart and lungs. Any other sites of symptoms should also be carefully examined for the reassurance of all concerned. In the breathless, a peak flow reading is helpful.

An attack of panic or hyperventilation is physiologically very demanding and cannot be sustained for more than a few minutes. This is perhaps as well since treatments for the acute episode are of limited effectiveness. Even an intravenous injection of a tranquilliser will take several minutes to work. The *air of calm and confidence* imparted by the GP is probably the most effective remedy. When the dust has settled, it is important to establish whether there is a history of similar events, or evidence of underlying anxiety or depression. Since treatment of any underlying cause will tend to be prolonged, and will often require insight by the patient, this may safely be left to an early follow-up appointment.

Managing chronic anxiety

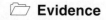 **Evidence**

The prognosis of chronic anxiety is not very good.

> **Prognosis[20]**
>
> A small study from general practice of non-psychotic psychiatric illness (mainly anxiety and depression) followed up over 11 years found that
>
> • Sufferers are twice as likely to die
> • Sufferers consult an average of 10 times a year
> • 50% have ongoing physical or mental illness
> • Most are treated only with medication.

It is necessary to spend sufficient time at the first consultation to establish the diagnosis, and to lay the foundations of a management plan. Most patients with anxiety do not consult a doctor at all, and so it might be supposed (but not proven) that those who do present have more debilitating symptoms. Many will have had their problem for a number of years.

What are the symptoms? This information will be readily forthcoming as it is uppermost in the patient's mind. When you hear the phrase; 'I don't know where to start', then you can usually assume that the patient is depressed or anxious, or both. A description of the symptoms will give a good idea of the diagnosis, and will usually reveal whether or not there are phobic, obsessional or panic elements to the anxiety.

Is there significant stress, or has there been an important life event? The death of a close relative or friend will always cause anxiety, especially in the early days, and this is not pathological. The search for lesser stresses is more problematic since most people appear to consider themselves under stress most of the time. The identification of *perceived life stresses* will, however, help to explain the symptoms and confirm that they do not represent a life-threatening disease.

Could there be a physical reason for the symptoms? Consumption of drugs, caffeine and alcohol should be enquired into. A *thyroid function* test is usually a good idea. Any other tests and investigations should only be ordered if there is a good chance of a helpful result. Since many anxious patients are already worried about their physical health, the ordering of the test and the wait for the results can cause further worry.

What is on the patient's agenda? Many will suspect that their symptoms are a result of anxiety, but at the same time do not want a physical diagnosis to be missed. To most people, the existence of a pain means that there is some tissue damage going on. Even if the patient is sure that the pain is being brought on by anxiety, there may yet be fear that damage is being caused as a result of the pain. The understanding that emotional illness can cause physical symptoms without physical damage is not widespread.[21]

There may be concern over *specific illnesses*, and the best way to find out about such concerns is to ask. Some patients will be reluctant to offer their concerns for fear of looking foolish, or because they are perplexed that the doctor is not automatically sharing their concerns. Appropriate questioning in such areas requires a high level of consulting skill.

What is expected from treatment? Medication is of limited use in treating anxiety disorders, and where it is useful there may be several weeks' delay before improvement is seen. A 'quick fix' solution is not usually possible. The best treatments are of the 'talking' type. Anyone undergoing such treatment must:

- Believe that the treatment is worth a try
- Take appropriate *responsibility* for the illness
- Be prepared to invest the right time and effort
- Be aware that treatment may uncover things which have been deliberately forgotten
- Sometimes be prepared to work in a group.

Treatment options

Treatments for anxiety fall into two main categories: medication and 'talking treatments' such as counselling and behavioural therapy. These are discussed below.

Before treatment of the anxiety begins, there are a few other jobs for the GP to do:

- *Exclude* physical disease
- *Explain* the basis of the symptoms. A discussion of the role of adrenaline and the 'fight or flight' reflex is usually helpful. For hyperventilation, a discussion of the physiological effects of overbreathing may help. For some, a leaflet will help, for instance the World Health Organisation have a series of leaflets available at a website which can be printed out in the surgery: www.psychiatry.ox.ac.uk/cebmh/whoguidemhpcuk/index.html
- Use *appropriate authority*. Many people who are anxious want someone to 'lean on' psychologically. This may be one of the few appropriate uses of medical authority.

Using medication

The use of medication is an attractive option in the management of anxiety. It is the most *accessible* type of treatment, and often brings about at least short-term relief of the symptoms. The drawback is that medication is rarely the best solution, and is often completely ineffective.

Benzodiazepines are very useful in acute anxiety, work quickly, have few somatic side effects, and are relatively safe in overdosage. There are, however, considerable problems with long-term use. There is still a role for benzodiazepines in the management of acute disabling anxiety, especially as a result of an acute stress. Diazepam 5 to 10 mg three times a day is about right, though it is best to use the *smallest effective dose*.

Buspirone does not seem to cause the dependency associated with the benzodiazepines. The onset of action is slow and progressive, and there is reduced efficacy in patients who have previously used benzodiazepines. Side effects include dizziness, headache and nausea. Sedation is minimal, and there is no interaction with alcohol. Cost is a problem.

Beta blockers may be effective in treating the *physical manifestations* of anxiety such as tremor, palpitations and sweating. Side effects include vivid dreams, tiredness and cold extremities. Propranolol 10 to 40 mg three times a day can be used.

Antidepressants. Imipramine, amitriptyline and clomipramine are beneficial in panic disorder. Clomipramine also has a licence for use in phobic and obsessive compulsive disorder.[13] In cases where anxiety is *mixed* with depression, or where the anxiety symptoms are an expression of underlying depression, the use of tricyclics is particularly beneficial. Problems of anticholinergic side effects, danger of overdose, and slow onset of action still apply, and the doses used are as for depression: e.g. imipramine 75 to 200 mg a day in divided doses.

All the selective serotonin re-uptake inhibitors are useful in panic disorder at the same doses as those used in depression. Other antidepressants such as mianserin and lofepramine are of *unproved* benefit in anxiety. They have fewer side effects but are more expensive.

Major tranquillisers in low doses can be used acutely and chronically in the treatment of anxiety. Problems include autonomic symptoms, restlessness and tardive dyskinesia.

Anithistamines are highly sedative and do not work.[8]

Psychological treatments

It is quite possible for a GP personally to offer a wide range of psychological therapies. Indeed the consultations which GPs have with the anxious will often make use of established psychological techniques, even if these techniques are not recognised as such. Picking up on patient cues, especially non-verbal cues, and then reflecting them back to a patient is a very powerful technique for getting psychological distress out into the open: 'I notice you clench your fist when you mention your father'. Each time a GP offers encouragement, a bit of supportive counselling or even cognitive therapy is going on.

To do the job properly, however, requires *training and sufficient time*, and most GPs will therefore choose to use outside experts for the more involved psychological treatments. Many GPs now employ counsellors in the practice, or are able to provide community psychiatric nurse (CPN) services at the surgery. When referring a patient on for such treatment it is important to have an idea what the treatment involves, so that you can tell the patient what to expect, and the patient can choose whether to accept such a treatment.

📁 **Evidence**

> **Effectiveness of psychological treatments**
>
> - About half your patients with anxiety disorders will regain a normal level of functioning after psychological treatment[22]
> - The less severely affected do better.[8]

Counselling involves discussion with the patient, and sometimes their family, and aims to help the patient use their existing personal resources to deal with the symptoms of anxiety and resolve any life problems. A typical course of treatment is six one-hour sessions at weekly intervals. Sometimes benefit continues with more prolonged courses.

In '*directive counselling*', specific sources of anxiety are identified, and the patient is encouraged (directed) to tackle them. This may require changes in the patient's lifestyle, relationships or even employment. At least four or five 15-minute sessions are required.[8]

Cognitive therapy is based on the observation that anxious people have anxious thoughts which prolong the anxious symptoms. Therapy aims to replace anxious attitudes, beliefs and images with more realistic variants. For example the patient with panic disorder may feel during an attack that death is imminent. Such a belief is wrong, and only serves to worsen the anxiety. Cognitive therapy is probably the most effective psychological treatment available for the anxiety disorders generally.[22]

Behavioural therapy aims to teach patients to replace maladaptive ways of coping. It is particularly useful in treating phobias where *graded exposure* may be used: a plan is agreed whereby the sufferer is exposed to progressively stronger phobic stimuli. Each stimulus is endured until the symptoms produced have abated, and the patient has learned that they can survive the experience. For instance, the grades used for a patient with agoraphobia may begin with getting the patient to imagine they are in a crowd, followed by walks in the street, visits to local shops, trips on the bus and finally attending a crowded occasion.

Applied relaxation. Anxiety causes muscle tension, and relaxing muscles is a good way of dissipating anxiety. The patient is encouraged to tense and then relax different muscle groups in a sequential manner. Most of the commercially available relaxation audio-tapes include a variety of this technique. A variant of this can be applied in acutely anxious situations. Suggest that the patient stand on one leg. Such is the concentration necessary to maintain balance that the anxiety is forgotten. More severe symptoms require the non-standing foot to be lifted higher.

Assertiveness training is currently very popular for all sorts of psychological problems. The therapist attempts to broaden the repertoire of the patient's responses in an inhibited interpersonal relationship.

Anxiety management is a package of different strategies combined for use with an individual patient. It may include some cognitive therapy, coping strategies and relaxation. Similar packages may be appropriate for different patients, and may well reflect the techniques with which the therapist has previously had good results.

Referral

Nearly all anxiety which is presented to a doctor is managed in primary care.[22] This will include the minor degrees of anxiety which are associated with ill health of any kind: if the patient wasn't worried about the symptoms, then presumably he or she would not bother consulting a doctor at all. Most GAD is also managed in primary care.

🗎 Guidelines

Specialist referral for anxiety[8,9]

- Severe symptoms
- Complicating psychological, social or physical problems
- Possible underlying physical cause
- Not responding to treatment
- Treatment needed which is not available in the community.

Summary

- It is normal and useful to react to stress
- At any time one in twenty people are experiencing anxiety, and over half have such symptoms in a given year
- Less than half of people with anxiety consult a doctor
- There are different sorts of anxiety, and their response to treatment differs
- Most anxiety which reaches medical attention is treated in primary care. Non-judgemental support, a cornerstone of normal general practice consulting, can result in therapeutic advantages. Nevertheless, anxiety is a chronic condition
- In anxiety, medication is little better than placebo except in acute anxiety. The long-term use of tranquillisers can be helpful, but there is concern about adverse side effects
- In the relatively common instance where depression and anxiety co-exist, the use of antidepressant medication often helps the anxiety and the depression
- The effective 'talking treatments' for anxiety require time, training for the therapist and considerable commitment from the patient.

🗩 Topics for discussion

- Stress and anxiety are inevitable components of life in the modern world
- The prescription of anxiolytics can never be justified
- A good GP will see anxious patients as often and for as long as the patient wants
- If you can't stand the heat, you should get out of the kitchen.

📖 References

1. RCGP (1986) Morbid statistics from general practice. Royal College of General Practitioners, Office of Population Censuses and Surveys, and Department of Health and Social Security. Third national study, 1981–82. London: HMSO.
2. Bullock T. Anxiety. *General Practitioner*, August 18, 1995; pp. 29–32.
3. McCartney D. The anxious patient. *Update* 1995; 51: 183–4.
4. Schryer J. Non-pharmacological management of anxiety. *Update* 1994; 48: 796–801.
5. Forte V J C. Management of anxiety disorders. *Update* 1999; 58; 533–7.
6. Life Change Index, *J. Psychosomatic Res.* 1967; 11: 213–8.
7. Bruce M S and Lader M. Caffeine: clinical experimental effects in humans. *Hum Psychopharmacol*, 1986; 1: 63–82.
8. Lader M. Treatment of anxiety. *BMJ* 1994; 309: 321–4.
9. Goldberg D, Bridges K, Duncan-Jones P et al. Detecting anxiety and depression in general medical settings. *BMJ*, 1988; 297: 897–9.
10. Davis M. Anxiety. *Update* 1998; 57: 411–13.
11. Power K G, Simpson R J, Swanson V et al. A controlled comparison of cognitive-behaviour therapy, diazepam, and placebo, alone and in combination, for the treatment of generalised anxiety disorder. *J Anxiety Dis* 1990; 4: 267–92.
12. Drug and Therapeutics. Psychological treatment for anxiety – an alternative to drugs? *Drug and Therapeutics Bulletin* 1993; 31: 73–5.
13. Tyrer P. Treating panic. *BMJ* 1989; 298: 201–2.
14. Sheenan D V. Benzodiazepines in panic disorder and agoraphobia. *J Affect Disord* 1987; 13: 169–81.
15. BMA. British National Formulary Number 41 (March), 2001; London: BMA/RPSGP.
16. Klosko J S, Barlow D H, Tassinari R et al. A comparison of alprazolam and behavior therapy in treatment of panic disorder. *J Consult Clin Psychol* 1990; 58: 77–84.
17. Marks I. Phobias and related anxiety disorder. *BMJ* 1991; 302:1037–8.
18. Jacobsen N S, Wilson L and Tupper C. The clinical significance of treatment gains resulting from exposure-based interventions for agoraphobia: a reanalysis of outcome data. *Behav Ther* 1988; 19: 539–44.
19. Wilkinson G. Stress, *General Practitioner* November 5, 1993; 43–8.
20. Lloyd K R, Jenkins R and Mann A. Long term outcome of patients with neurotic illness in general practice. *BMJ* 1996; 313: 26–8.
21. Boardman J. Detection of psychological problems by general practitioners. *Update* 1991; 42, 1067–3.
22. Durham R C and Allen T. Psychological treatment of generalised anxiety disorder. A review of the clinical significance of results in outcome studies since 1980. *Br J Psychiatry* 1993; 163: 19–26.

Behaviour problems in children

Tutorial aim

The registrar can respond appropriately to abnormal childhood behaviour.

Learning objectives

By the end of the tutorial the registrar can:

- List three features of hyperactivity
- List three features of autism
- List four features of dyslexia
- Prescribe appropriately in encopresis
- Discuss the effects of abnormal childhood behaviour on the rest of the family
- With parents and child refer appropriately
- Compose an appropriate referral letter
- Describe a programme of behaviour modification for a child.

Preliminaries

At least from time to time, all parents are caused anxiety by the behaviour of their children. Problem behaviour is always a *two way process*: the nature of the behaviour, and the response of the parents. It is invariably the child who is presented as the patient with the problem, but the child's behaviour cannot be understood without also understanding how other family members may be contributing. This is not to suggest, however, that the child's behaviour is the fault of the parents. It is important that the parents are not alienated: their cooperation is vital if treatment is to succeed. Some parents will *tolerate* very disruptive behaviour. This tolerance may give a significant insight into why the behaviour is occurring.

Behaviour must be seen in the context of the *developmental age* of the child. Selfish behaviour at the age of two is normal, but at twelve is unacceptable. This will often make problem behaviour at least understandable, if not tolerable. Stress or other illness may make a child retreat to a former developmental stage and so exhibit behaviour appropriate to that stage: *regression*.

A general practitioner or health visitor will often be called upon to give advice on the appropriate management of minor behavioural problems. In *rare* instances the behaviour occurs as a result of a more serious disorder. If there is any doubt about one of these more severe diagnoses, specialist assessment and help should be secured at an early stage. All children are different. Even between siblings there may be major differences in temperament. Professionals and carers outside the family may be more aware of the *range of normal* behaviour seen in this age group, and will be able to reassure parents accordingly.[1] Particularly in younger children, the *health visitor* is an important ally for GP and parents. Health visitors have sufficient training and experience of normal child development to take on many of the problems encountered. For older children there is a clear role for the school nursing service.

Changing child behaviour

🗎 Guidelines

Elements of effective discipline[2]

- A learning environment characterised by positive supportive parent–child relationships
- A strategy for systematic teaching and strengthening of desired behaviours
- A strategy for decreasing or eliminating undesired behaviours.

A positive learning environment is one in which parents take an *interest* in what the child does, *praise* acceptable behaviour, *encourage* the child to take part in the life of the household, *allow choices*, and are sensitive to the child's developmental *needs* and emotional responses to stress. Desired behaviour can be reinforced by rewards.

Difficult behaviour may either be ignored or may lead to some sort of penalty. Suitable penalties might be the removal of parental *attention* for a specified number of minutes, or (particularly in older children) the withdrawal of privileges. Children thrive on routine and consistency: behavioural *boundaries* should be set and kept to. The use of penalties should be explained to the child, and should be appropriate to the offence.

Most families in the UK use physical punishments to discipline their children. This seems to be an effective way of making the child behave better in the immediate aftermath of the punishment, but does not result in the learning of desired behaviour.[2]

Under fives

Temper tantrums

The usual age is eighteen months to three years.[1] Tantrums are only effective if there is an audience. If the child is put in a safe place and left alone, and the tantrum not referred to again, then this method of getting attention rapidly loses its appeal. Temper tantrums do not cause fits or brain haemorrhage. If they are associated with severe breath holding there may be a temporary loss of consciousness, but generally the child is vividly aroused during the episode.

Tantrums are invariably preceded by a *stimulus* of some sort, and the agitation runs an *escalating course* before the main event of the full-blown tantrum. If the description of the tantrum suggests a seizure then this should be investigated, but otherwise treatment is by explanation and advice to the parents on how to cope.

Food refusal

A child cannot be forced to eat. Eating refusal causes particular parental anxiety as there is the additional concern that the poor eating will lead to ill health. Weighing the child to demonstrate that no harm is resulting is a good way of alleviating anxiety. Very rarely there is a genuine and consistent failure to gain weight, and in such cases a more severe problem or even the extremely rare example of childhood anorexia nervosa should be remembered. Sensible advice includes[1]

- Make mealtimes peaceful and free of tension. Wait till the siblings are at school
- At first give small meals on a small plate
- Parents and other family members should not comment on how little the child is eating
- After reasonable encouragement, remove the meal and don't offer food till the next meal time
- Make sure the child is receiving attention between meals in socially acceptable ways.

Bowel problems

Encopresis is defined as 'faecal soiling by children after the point at which bowel control should have been achieved and for which no underlying organic cause is responsible'.[3] To fit the diagnosis the soiling should occur at least *once a month*. The typical starting age is three or four, and the prevalence is 2 to 3% of boys and 0.7% of girls at age seven, falling to half this at age eleven.[3]

It has been estimated that in 90% of cases a common path is followed: withholding of faeces causes megacolon with overflow and soiling.[3] The distended colon is insensitive to feelings of fullness.

In some cases the child withholds faeces because of conflict within the family or because of deep psychological trauma: the child may also show slowed intellectual development. In other cases domestic life is inconsistent and chaotic so that no toilet routine is established. Whatever the psychological or family pathology underlying the encopresis, it should also be remembered that in a majority of cases the child gets *pain on defecation*:[3] the pain needs treatment as well.

The first step in treatment is to get the colon cleared. Once pain-free defecation is established the encopresis will often right itself. This can be done with laxatives, but sometimes enemas are needed or manual clearance. Once a normal bowel habit has been established the laxative can be withdrawn, but this should be done *gradually* over months. Causes of pain on defecation, such as *fissures*, should be attended to. A toilet routine should be established if not already present, and some children respond well to *star charts* and other reward methods. The children who do not respond or who show signs of developmental delay or psychological illness will need referring.

Sleep problems

During childhood the pattern of sleep changes markedly. The *cycle* of deep to shallow sleep takes 90 minutes in an adult, but only 47 minutes in the newborn.[4] All young children wake repeatedly through the night: the trick is to get them to go to sleep again without disturbing the household.

Sleep problems often start at around two years. This is just the time when the birth of a sibling is most likely: the parents will be coping with a newborn baby at the same time as the sleeping problem. By age three, 15% of children have a sleep disturbance, and 10% are still having problems at age eight.[5] A problem with sleeping is the most common infant behavioural disorder presented to the GP.

An approach to a sleep problem might include

- *History*: the problem may be of frequent waking, trouble getting to sleep, or both
- *Examine*: this is to rule out any physical reason for the sleep problem. Children in pain are unable to sleep
- *Parental reaction*: sleep problems are rarely caused by parents, but the way parents react can influence their course. All children wake, but if they are always cuddled back to sleep then they lose the ability to fall asleep uncuddled
- *Assessment of parents*: are they exhausted? Are they worried that some harm will befall their child because of sleeplessness? Is there concern about an illness? Is there guilt because the parents feel the problem results from their lack of parenting skills?

Problems falling asleep can usually be tackled by the establishment of a definite bedtime *routine*. A sequence such as bath, then story, then drink, then cuddle, then to bed, will establish the normality of going to sleep. The delay between announcing that it is bedtime and getting the child into bed should not be either excessively long or of variable length. If bedtime needs to be brought forward, this can be done gradually with bedtime getting 15 minutes earlier every 2 or 3 nights.

Repeated waking is best tackled by a phased *withdrawal of attention* from the crying child. This is hard as parents are biologically doomed to feel awful if their baby is crying. Each time the child cries in the night, the parent attends after an increased delay, and stays for a decreased time. The delays and time with the child will need to be worked out beforehand, and then timed with a clock: it is easy to imagine the child has been crying for hours. Such a programme is exhausting, and it may be several nights before a result is achieved, so it is important that the parents share the work. Some hardy parents will try to get it over with by not attending the child at all. This can work, but the neighbours should be warned. Other parents find that getting the child in bed with them makes for peace and quiet. This is a bit 'un-English' but can be effective, and in many cultures is the accepted norm:

worldwide more women sleep with their children than with their husbands.[4]

Nightmares: where the child wakes remembering a bad dream, are usually self-limiting. *Night terrors* happen during deeper sleep, and are not remembered. The child is distressed but still asleep and unresponsive. An older age group is involved, and problems may persist for years. The terrors often occur at the same time each night, so one useful strategy is to wake the child before the terror happens.

Five to eleven years

Behavioural problems in the five- to eleven-year-olds are *less common*, but tend to be harder to deal with. In most cases treatment will be necessary. Difficulties are usually the result of *wider pathology within the family*, but occasionally occur because of significant pathology within the child. Some disorders, especially if severe, will be diagnosed before the age of five, but will continue to require management throughout the early school years.

About one in ten children aged five to fifteen have a mental disorder

- 5% conduct disorder
- 4% emotional disorder
- 1% hyperkinetic disorder.

There is a steep social class gradient, so that children in social class V have three times the disorder rate of those in social class I. Children whose parents have never worked have a 20% risk of disorder.[6] Global learning delay is often found to co-exist.

A practical approach

The GP will have prior knowledge of the child and the other family members. Time should be spent in *establishing the facts* of each case: even if a referral is needed the GP can often provide useful background information and will want to stay in touch with progress. The health visitor should also be involved, and may well have further information to contribute.

What are the symptoms? Details of the problem behaviour should be sought. An 'A, B, C' analysis can be useful

- what are the Antecedents?
- of what nature is the Behaviour?
- what are the Consequences?

Does the behaviour happen in all circumstances, or only at home or at school? Are there any learning difficulties co-existing? Is there an abnormally short attention span?

How do the parents react? The parents may have their own problems, such as depression or learning difficulties, which are making it *difficult to cope*. There may be poor support from relatives and friends, particularly in single parent households. Parental tolerance may be lower than average: parents may over-react to some types of behaviour, such as aggression, or they may have formed their expectations of behaviour from an older child who has a different temperament. How hard are the parents willing to work to bring about an improvement in the child's behaviour? Their cooperation is vital for success.

Are there family stresses? Strains within the marriage may cause, or indeed be the consequence of, difficult child behaviour. Some families lack appropriate *parenting skills* with respect to giving the child attention and reacting to problem behaviour. There may have been a separation or death in the family which everyone is reacting to.

What are home circumstances like? Problem behaviour is commoner in overcrowded and deprived households. There may be insufficient space and toys for play. Play may not be adequately supervised. There may be too much or too little contact with adults and other children. During childhood more time is spent watching *television* than in the classroom.[8] Some vulnerable children learn aggressive behaviour as a way of solving problems, and once learned these habits are very difficult to modify. In some cases the images received from the television contribute to aggressive behaviour, and may provoke anxiety and fear. However for the majority of children occasional viewing is unlikely to have an adverse effect.[7]

Aggression

This is one of the most troubling childhood behaviour disorders and is found in 4% of rural populations and 9% of urban populations. Around a third of GP consultations with children and nearly half those with community child health services are for behavioural problems.[8] The behaviour of which the parents complain is usually an exaggeration of commonly found traits. The problem may be either one of degree, or of parental tolerance. The types of behaviour encountered may include

- Disobedience, tantrums, occasional aggression and high levels of activity at home
- Disruption in the classroom and aggression towards other children. There may be a global learning disorder, and a third have reading problems[8]
- At age six, children can usually distinguish between their property and that of others: stealing and lying may occur
- Running away from home, engaging in dangerous activities, truancy.

About 40% of aggressive seven- and eight-year-olds become *delinquent* adolescents.[8] The amount of crime committed by children under eighteen is certainly increasing. The threat of punishment will deter the occasional offender, but seems to have little effect on the committed juvenile criminal.[9] At age eight the best predictors of subsequent offending are:[9]

- Hyperactivity, impulsivity, and attention deficit
- Marital discord between the child's parents
- Harsh or erratic parenting
- Socio-economic deprivation

- Separation from the parents for reasons other than death or illness.

These factors seem to be additive.

Aggressive children are *usually unhappy*. Typically they have poor social skills and few friends. Self-esteem is poor. School achievement is below average – the typical IQ is around 10 points below that of contemporaries.[8]

Treatment requires specialised assessment and implementation. Individual psychotherapy does not work, but behaviourally-based programmes to help parents have consistently been shown to be effective.[8] A typical programme is ten sessions. Children from high-risk families can be helped not to offend by training in social skills, and their parents benefit from being taught parenting skills.

Somatising

This is defined as *psychological distress giving rise to physical symptoms.*[10]

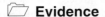 **Evidence**

Prevalence of somatised symptoms[10]

- Commonest symptoms are headache and abdominal pain
- Of school age children 10% have recurrent abdominal pain
- Of children attending a general paediatric clinic 50% have somatised symptoms
- Of children attending their GP 20% will have a psychological problem which is making their symptoms worse
- Only 5% of children referred to a specialist with abdominal pain will have a serious physical illness.

Though uncommon, it is necessary to *rule out physical pathology* before family anxiety can be relieved and a psychological diagnosis agreed. A discussion of the physical effects of psychological illness, and uncovering possible sources of stress from the history can both be useful ways of making progress with the child and family.

Children with recurrent abdominal pains tend to be conformist, eager to gain approval and sensitive to distress and insecurity. There has often been a recent excess of significant life events such as deaths, exams, etc. Somatising disorders in the parents are associated with an excess of unexplained physical disorders in their children.[10]

The overall health of the child will reassure the GP that a serious physical diagnosis is not being missed. Using a diagnosis like *abdominal migraine* may actually be true, and if not at least serves to emphasise the fact that the pain does not signify a serious physical disorder. The majority of children *improve with time*. There is a reduction in the frequency of the attacks, and either a reduction in severity or a reduction in the alarm caused by the pain.

An *explanation* of the disorder should be helpful and make the symptoms less worrying to child and parents. Specific stress management techniques may help, but these are probably best left to the child psychiatry services.

A recent sudden onset of a psychosomatic disorder may indicate *sexual abuse*.

Symptoms may be confounded by problems with *school refusal* so that the child is regularly kept from school because of the symptoms. In such cases it may be impossible to establish which is the primary disorder, and so treatment is needed for each.

Hearing loss

Sensorineural hearing loss in children is rare and usually congenital. The usual cause of conductive loss is secretory otitis media (*glue ear*) and it is estimated that up to 80% of children have at least one episode of this in their lives.[11]

Glue ear is commoner in boys and peaks at ages three to six years. Hearing loss is often the only symptom, and is commonly suspected first by the parents. If they report concern about their child's hearing, this should be taken very seriously whatever the lack of other evidence to support the diagnosis.

Hearing loss causes children perceptual and expressive problems. The inability to take in information accurately leads to confusion, frustration and anger. Children who are unable to hear instructions are unable to please their parents and so fail to gain approval. Different types of behaviour are tried in order to get a response. Expressive problems are caused by the poor development of language which is a consequence of not being able to hear others speak. Non-verbal communication is therefore attempted, and behavioural changes result.

Up to half of all children with a hearing deficit will display *behavioural problems*.[11] Those most frequently seen are overactivity, short attention span, poor relations with other children, temper tantrums and being out of parental control. Longer-term problems include conduct disorders which last to adolescence, subtle language deficits, poorer educational attainment, persisting difficulties with relationships and long-term effects on self-esteem and self-confidence.

Audiometry is an accurate and non-invasive procedure. Any child in whom there is suspicion of a hearing deficit, especially if there are behavioural problems, should be properly tested.

Hyperactivity

The establishment of a diagnosis of hyperactivity is fraught with problems

- Normal children have loads of energy
- Definitions of hyperactivity differ from country to country
- Schools may be reluctant to accept the diagnosis because the *statementing* of a child has financial implications
- The use of methylphenidate (Ritalin) is hotly debated and may be subject to *post-code rationing*
- There may be concern over the contribution of food additives.

The main features of hyperactivity fall into three areas[12]

- Inattention
- Overactivity
- Impulsiveness.

Examples of typical behaviour are given in the box. The problematic behaviour must be present in *more than one setting*. Problems in a single area constitute *Attention Deficit Hyperactivity Disorder* (ADHD). When a child has problems in all three behavioural areas, then the diagnosis is of *Hyperkinetic Disorder* (HKD).

📄 **Guidelines**

Features of hyperactivity[13]

- *Inattention*:

    forgetful, loses things, distractable
    inattention to detail, doesn't finish things
    unable to sustain attention, seems not to listen
    unable to organise things

- *Overactivity*:

    fidgets, always 'on the go'
    leaps out of seat, runs about and climbs
    can't play quietly, talks a lot

- *Impulsivity*:

    unable to wait
    interrupts, blurts out the answers.

The prevalence of ADHD is 3 to 5%, and of HKD 0.5 to 1%. Parents and teachers think the prevalence of ADHD is 24%.[13] Children with hyperkinetic disorder are at considerable developmental risk and have high rates of motor and language delay.[14] In 50% there is also another psychological or physical problem.[13] Sufferers are prone to develop anti-social conduct disorders. Severe hyperactivity may continue into adolescence and adult life, but between half and two thirds of children 'grow out' of HKD or ADHD by the teenage years.[13]

Assessment and treatment should be under *specialist supervision*. Behaviour modification and special education are the mainstays of treatment. Some,[12] but by no means all hyperactive children[15] will benefit from *dietary modification*. Often several foods are implicated: the simple exclusion of food additives is unlikely to achieve the desired result. The use of stimulants such as methylphenidate is associated with improved behaviour.[16]

Autism

The *autistic spectrum* is a group of developmental disorders characterised by problems in three areas

- Social interaction
- Communication
- Imagination.

The spectrum includes autism (described in 1943) and Asperger's syndrome (described in 1944). It is possibly brought on by organic brain damage in early years,[17] but it is certainly not the result of emotional trauma or poor parenting.

Autism affects around 5 per 10 000 children severely, and a further 20 per 10 000 have autistic tendencies. It is a rare disorder which an average GP will see only once every 80 years. The overall prevalence of the autistic spectrum is 91 per 10 000.[18]

Autism often accompanies other developmental disorders, and four boys are affected for every girl. Of those diagnosed, 10% will be able to live independently, 30% will need some support and the rest will be significantly handicapped and completely dependent.[17]

Guidelines

National Autistic Society – Aids to diagnosis[19]

Sufferers may

- Show what they want by using an adult's hand
- Parrot a question instead of answering it
- Laugh or giggle, often for no reason
- Talk incessantly about one topic
- Exhibit bizarre behaviour
- Handle or spin objects
- Avoid eye contact
- Avoid creative play but order objects repetitively
- Join in games with other children only if adults insist
- Be able to do tasks quickly so long as they don't involve social interaction
- Do some things very well, but not those involving social understanding.

The diagnosis is usually made by age three. *Parental observations* are of greatest importance. The role of the GP is to be suspicious and refer on for proper assessment. The child and carers will need extra support while a diagnosis is being reached formally, and thereafter as the long-term effects of the disorder become apparent. Most autistic children cannot be handled within the normal school system, and there is often a high level of involvement with the local Department of Social Services over care and respite.

Dyslexia

Dyslexia is a learning disorder causing difficulty with reading, spelling and writing despite *average or above average intelligence* and normal schooling. A subgroup have specific difficulty with spelling – dysgraphia. Other problems may be an inability to read music or difficulty with mathematics.

Depending on the diagnostic criteria used,[20] 4 to 10% of children are affected Four boys are affected for each girl. There is evidence of *genetic transmission*. There may be an overlap with ADHD, or with minor neurological disorders causing clumsiness or unsteady gait. Other sufferers may become shy and withdrawn.[21] The features of dyslexia include

- Late speech development
- Difficulty labelling known objects or remembering people's names

- Persistent word searching
- Excessive 'spoonerisms'
- Difficulty learning nursery rhymes, days of the week, months of the year, etc.
- Often clumsy
- Difficulty throwing, catching or kicking a ball, or with hopping, skipping and clapping rhythms
- Late learning to fasten buttons
- Continuing to put shoes on the wrong feet in spite of the discomfort.

The job of the GP if dyslexia is suspected is to refer on to an *educational psychologist* for full assessment and management. Treatment is by special educational techniques. The sooner the condition is recognised and treatment begun, the less disruption is caused to the child's development.

Developmental dyspraxia

Some children show difficulties in motor coordination out of proportion to their other general abilities. Balance or frequent falls may be a problem. There may be problems with speech or writing. Males are more commonly affected. A clumsy child may be bullied and have low self-esteem. This may lead to abnormal behaviour in other spheres, withdrawal or psychosomatic aches and pains. Physiotherapy, occupational therapy and special educational techniques can all help.

Guidelines

Detection of developmental dyspraxia[22]

test:

- Heel-to-toe walking across the room
- Walking on tiptoe
- Standing on one leg for eight seconds
- Unscrewing jar lid (should manage by two years)
- Building a tower of five bricks.

School refusal

On any one day, 10% of children are absent from school, but only 1 to 2% are away because of school refusal.[23] School attendance is required by the Education Act 1981, and the Children Act 1989 contains powers to supervise any child whose school attendance is poor. It is not unusual for school refusal to present as *physical symptoms* with no obvious cause. Typical somatised symptoms include

- Nausea
- Abdominal pain
- Headache
- 'Wobbly legs'.

There are four categories of children who do not attend school

- *School refusal* is when all parental efforts to get the child to school are resisted. It is likely to be a continuing problem

- *Truancy* is when the child misses school without the knowledge of the parents. It tends to be a group activity
- *School phobia* is when the child is overwhelmingly frightened of some aspect of the school, and so will not attend
- *Withholding* is where the parents collude to keep the child from school. The parents may want the child at home either because of fears over the child's health, or because of their own psychological needs.

Bullying is widespread in schools with over a quarter of junior school children affected.[24] Bullied children have lower self-esteem, lack confidence and have fewer close friends. Schoolwork may suffer. There is an increase in headaches, tummy aches, bedwetting, sleep difficulties, and feelings of sadness.[24] Bullied children are more likely as adults to suffer anxiety, depression and loneliness, and may also have trouble with heterosexual relationships.[24] Tactful questions to explore whether or not the child feels bullied are an important part of fact-finding when problem behaviour is presented. Having established the facts, the GP will wish to involve the teacher and the educational welfare officer, and possibly the educational psychologist. It is usually appropriate to organise a gentle graduated re-exposure to the school environment.

Summary

- Childhood behavioural disorders are common and always involve the rest of the family
- Most problems in the under-fives can be solved by the application of sensible parenting advice. Health visitors are particularly good at this
- Medication for constipation works, medication for sleep problems usually does not
- Developmental, behavioural and learning problems often co-exist
- Hyperactivity is diagnosed more often by parents and teachers than it is by psychologists
- The prognosis for complete recovery from hyperactivity is up to 70%
- Autism has a very poor prognosis for independent life
- Minor degrees of dyslexia are relatively common, and respond well to special educational techniques. Early diagnosis is therefore crucial
- Even for problems insoluble in primary care, a GP still has a responsibility for gathering evidence and referring appropriately. Sufferers from the more severe conditions, and their families, will need ongoing support
- Don't forget hearing loss as a possible cause of difficult child behaviour.

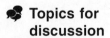 Topics for discussion

Address the implications behind the following statements:

- Strange parents raise strange children
- There is no law against smacking a child
- Parents are responsible for the behaviour of their children
- All children with behaviour problems should be referred to a specialist
- The health visitor or school nurse should be involved whenever a child displays problem behaviour.

📖 **References**

1. Cook N. Behaviour problems. *The Practitioner* 1993; 237: 687–91.
2. Waterston T. Giving guidance on child discipline. *BMJ* 2000; 320: 261–2.
3. McColl M. Tackling encopresis. *Medical Monitor* 1992; 5(39): 59–62.
4. Haslam D. 'My child won't sleep'. *The Practitioner* 1995; 239: 730–2.
5. McColl M. When sleeping beauties turn into beasts. *Medical Monitor* 1991; 4(22): 53–7.
6. Yamey G. Survey finds that 1 in 10 children has a mental disorder. *BMJ* 1999; 319: 1456.
7. Black D and Newman M. Television violence and children. *BMJ* 1995; 310: 273–4.
8. Scott S. Aggressive behaviour in childhood. *BMJ* 1998; 316: 202–6.
9. Shepherd J P and Farrington D P. Preventing crime and violence. *BMJ* 1995; 310: 271–2.
10. Garralda M E and Hughes T P. Worried sick – somatisation in children. *Maternal and Child Health* 1994; 19: 40–4.
11. Barber W, Griffiths M V and Williams R. Behaviour disorders and hearing loss in pre-school children. *Update* 1992; 44: 1132–40.
12. The management of hyperactive children. *Drug and Therapeutics Bulletin* 1995; 33: 57–60.
13. Cameron M L. Attention deficit disorder. *Update* 1998; 57: 512–5.
14. Taylor E and Hemsley R. Treating hyperkinetic disorder in childhood. *BMJ* 1995; 310: 1617–18.
15. Taylor E and Heptinstall E. Dietary treatment for hyperactivity – does it work? *Maternal and Child Health* 1990; 15: 98–102.
16. Zwi M, Ramchandani P and Joughin C. Evidence and belief in ADHD. *BMJ* 2000; 321: 975–6.
17. Plachta J. Be vigilant over bizarre behaviour. *General Practitioner* May 8 1992: 66.
18. Gould J. Autism. *General Practitioner* May 22 1998: 56–7.
19. Aids to Diagnosis of Autism. London: *National Autistic Society*, 1992.
20. Goulandris N, Newton A and Auger J. Dyslexia. *General Practitioner* December 4 1992: 43–8.
21. British Dyslexia Association. Dyslexia: A Guide for the Medical and Healthcare Professions. Reading: BDA, 1996.
22. Waterston T. Managing the clumsy and non-reading child. *The Practitioner* 1999; 243: 675–7.
23. McColl M. Children who won't go to school. *Medical Monitor* 1992; 5(8): 81–4.
24. Dawkins J. Bullying in schools: doctors' responsibilities. *BMJ* 1995; 310: 274–5.

Benign prostatic hypertrophy and prostate cancer

Tutorial aim	**The registrar is able to assess and manage mild to moderate male obstructive urinary outflow symptoms within primary care.**
Learning objectives	By the end of the tutorial the registrar can: • List five symptoms of bladder outflow obstruction (BOO) • Describe the initial assessment of a patient with BOO symptoms • Discuss with a patient the treatment options for benign prostatic hypertrophy (BPH) • Discuss the advantages and disadvantages of prostate surgery for BPH • Discuss with a patient and his family the implications of a diagnosis of prostate cancer • Discuss the evidence for and against screening for prostate cancer.

Preliminaries

The prostate is a wedge-shaped gland found only in males. It is made mainly of smooth muscle, and is situated at the base of the bladder, surrounding the urethra. The prostate grows with age from about 35 years onwards, so that at age 85 virtually all men will have evidence of enlargement.[1]

The terminology is confusing, benign prostatic enlargement (BPE) is the normal enlargement with age. Lower urinary tract symptoms (LUTS) is a term currently in vogue and refers to the symptoms which prostatic enlargement may cause. Bladder outflow obstruction (BOO) is the presumed cause of those symptoms. However, still the most widely used term among GPs is benign prostatic hypertrophy (BPH), which covers both the pathology and the symptoms of prostatic enlargement.

Each year in England and Wales around 15 000 men will be diagnosed with prostate cancer and 10 000 will die,[2] making it the second most common cause of death[3] from cancer. It is also a disease of increasing age, being twice as common in the ninth decade as in the seventh decade of life.[4] The incidence of new cases is rising fast, nearly doubling between 1971 and 1991,[2] even allowing for the facts that longevity is increasing and in some countries screening is detecting very early cases.[4] Prostate cancer is not causally related to BPH but the two conditions commonly coexist,[5] and signs and symptoms are often the same.

Signs and symptoms   The enlarging prostate obstructs urinary outflow. The bladder muscle reacts to this obstruction by becoming irritable. Symptoms are caused by the obstruction itself and also by the bladder irritability. Anything which causes BOO can give identical symptoms.

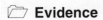 **Guidelines**   **Symptoms of bladder outflow obstruction**

- Caused by obstruction (*voiding symptoms*)

    hesitancy
    poor stream
    interrupted stream, double voiding
    terminal dribbling
    urinary retention

- Caused by bladder irritability (*filling symptoms*)

    nocturia
    feeling of incomplete voiding
    urgency
    dysuria
    frequency
    incontinence.

Evidence

> **Prevalence of BOO symptoms[6]**
>
> A community postal survey of 1500 men over 55 years living in North West Thames found that:
>
> - 20% had moderate or severe symptoms of BOO
> - 59% had mild symptoms
> - Only 21% had no symptoms at all
> - Prevalence of symptoms increased with age. Moderately/severely affected: aged 55 to 64 = 16%; 65 to 79 = 25%; over 85 = 12% (includes those who had had surgery).

- Around half of men with BOO find their symptoms 'troublesome',[7] and in a third to half of men with moderate or severe symptoms there is disruption of daily activities[6]
- Between 5 and 15% of men over 65 have two or more episodes of urinary incontinence a month[8]
- Hesitancy, urgency and dribbling are found to be most troublesome,[7] but most men over 60 regard these symptoms as a natural consequence of ageing. Pain, acute retention and haematuria are not regarded as normal[7]

- Under half of men with BOO symptoms consult a doctor because of them.[9] Men with moderate or severe symptoms are six times more likely to consult than those with mild symptoms,[9] but are no more likely to be referred to a urologist.

The *International Prostate Symptom Score (IPSS)* is a patient self-assessment tool from which the severity of bladder outflow obstruction can be assessed. It can be repeated during and after treatment to assess progress.

📄 **Guidelines**   **IPSS questions**[10]

For the first six questions:

Not at all	0
Less than one time in five	1
Less than half the time	2
About half the time	3
More than half the time	4
Almost always	5

1. Over the past month, how often have you had a sensation of not emptying your bladder completely after you have finished urinating?
2. Over the past month, how often have you had the urge to urinate again less than two hours after you last finished urinating?
3. Over the past month, how often have you found you stopped and started again several times when you urinated?
4. Over the past month, how often have you found it difficult to postpone urination?
5. Over the past month, how often have you had a weak urinary stream? (Please compare with your stream size at age 30).
6. Over the past month, how often have you had to push or strain to begin urination?
7. Over the past month, how many times did you typically get up to urinate from the time you went to bed at night until the time you got up in the morning?
   (Score never = 0, once = 1 etc., to five or more = 5)

Total Scores		
	Severe	20–35
	Moderate	8–19
	Mild	<8

The initial assessment

Prostate cancer and BPH both cause BOO, and the patient's symptoms are often identical. The aims of the initial assessment are, therefore

- Exclude cancer
- Look for secondary damage resulting from BOO.

📄 **Guidelines**   **Initial assessment of male BOO**[5]

The UK British Prostate Group and others recommend

'Full medical history', presumably for evidence of metastatic disease

Urinary symptom review
Digital rectal examination (DRE)
Urine analysis
Serum creatinine, for renal failure
It would also seem sensible to include an abdominal examination looking for
evidence of urinary retention.

Doing a DRE is the only way of physically examining the prostate. It is
unpleasant for both examiner and examinee, so its use should be justified. A
normal prostate has a firm, rubbery feel to it, and its architecture (specifically
the median sulcus) is usually palpable. It is only a crude way of assessing
prostatic volume, and anyway the severity of BOO symptoms is more closely
related to the patient's age than to prostatic volume.[11] Most prostate cancers
start in the periphery of the gland and so are, in theory, palpable. However,
the commonest prostate cancers are under 2 mm across, and these are unlikely
to be felt on DRE.[12]

The measurement of Prostate Specific Antigen (PSA) is not recommended as
a routine in all patients. It is, however, recommended if there is suspicion of
cancer, or if there is a family history of prostate cancer at under 75 years of
age.[5] Cancer is commoner in older patients, and in the presence of symptoms
such as haematuria and haematospermia. Patients with a history in first degree
relatives of prostate or breast cancer have a two to threefold increased risk of
prostate cancer.[13]

📂 **Evidence**

PSA levels[14]

- PSA levels are raised by:

    acute retention
    catheterisation
    prostatitis
    BPH
    prostate cancer

- And lowered by:

    5 alpha reductase inhibition
    ejaculation (85% reduction[15])

- PSA also varies with age

    40 to 49: under 2.5 ng/ml
    70 to 79: under 6.5 ng/ml

The level of PSA is not altered by DRE,[14] so it is all right to do the examination
and then decide if PSA estimation would be helpful. Doing a PSA without
DRE is not very helpful: around 40% of men with prostate cancer have a PSA
below 4 ng/ml.[16] A combination of DRE and a PSA over 4 ng/ml has 96%
sensitivity for prostate cancer,[17] but is not very specific.[4]

Management plan   If cancer is not suspected, then it is appropriate for the GP to have a go at treatment.

Watchful waiting   The symptoms of BOO do not inevitably get worse, and in many cases improve with time. The obstruction will not go away, but the bladder muscle may become more tolerant of its burden. Also, patients may become more tolerant of the symptoms either because they are genuinely less troubled, or because they have adjusted their lifestyle to cope.

📁 **Evidence**

Natural history of symptoms of BOO[18]

In a survey 1610 men in Stirling aged 40 to 79 with symptoms of BOO were followed up over 12 months

Symptoms unchanged	60 to 70%
Symptoms worse	10 to 20%
Symptoms improved	15 to 20%

Some men do not want treatment anyway. Such has been the publicity over prostate cancer that a reassurance that the gland is not malignant is all that is required. In other instances, a discussion of the possible treatment options will result in a decision to leave well alone, at least until such time as treatment might be an improvement over symptoms. About a fifth of men who consult their GP with BPH are *treated by reassurance*.[9]

Medication   *Alpha blockade* reduces sympathetic tone in the smooth muscles of the prostate and bladder. The bladder effects improve the *filling* symptoms of BOO, and the prostate effects improve the *voiding* symptoms. An improvement of urinary flow of between 30 and 40% can be expected,[19] but perhaps more significantly 80% of patients report symptomatic improvement which relapses if the treatment is stopped.[20] The treatment takes a week or two to work.

Side effects of alpha blockers include:

- First dose hypotension
- Weight gain
- Drowsiness
- Impotence
- Nasal congestion
- Dry mouth.

They should not be used in patients with heart failure, and should be used with caution in patients with impaired renal or hepatic function. There is nothing to choose between products in terms of efficacy or side effect profiles. The cheapest is prazosin which at a dose of 1 mg bd costs £35 a year.[21]

Finasteride is the only 5-alpha reductase inhibitor currently available in the UK. The drug reduces the circulating levels of dihydrotestosterone by up to

80%,[22] and this reduces the volume of the prostate by up to 28% after six months of treatment.[5] It seems to work best in men with very large prostates, of whom at least half can expect an improvement in symptoms.[5] Finasteride is usually well tolerated:

- Impotence 3.7%
- Low ejaculatory volume 2.9%
- Decreased libido 3.3%. However, coital frequency is anyway decreased in men with BPH symptoms.[22]

It is more expensive than prazosin: 5 mg a day for a year costs £325.[21]

Reasons to refer

Of the men who present to their GP with symptoms of BOO, about two thirds eventually get referred to a urologist.[9] The severity of symptoms does not seem to influence the decision to refer.[18] Anyone with suspected cancer needs urgent specialist assessment. Others who need to be seen promptly are those in whom there has been damage secondary to BOO, such as renal impairment or acute or chronic retention.

📄 Guidelines

Specialist referral[1]

Refer when:

- *Urgent*

    elevated creatinine or hydronephrosis
    haematuria
    suspicion of cancer: suspicious DRE, PSA over 4 ng/ml
    bladder or prostate pain
    confirmed urinary tract infection
    suspected urinary retention

- *Non-urgent*

    failure to respond to medical treatment
    severe symptoms

Men who are referred to a urologist because of BOO symptoms will be investigated by any or all of the following procedures

- Repeat initial assessment, as above
- Renal ultrasound
- Cystoscopy
- Uroflometry
- Prostatic biopsy
- Rectal ultrasound

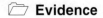 **Evidence**

> ### Outcome of specialist referral[9]
>
> As a result of seeing a urologist and undergoing further investigations
>
> - 79% of men are offered surgery, of whom 71% accept
> - 4% receive medication
> - 17% 'treated by reassurance'

Talking about Surgery

Surgery is the initial treatment preference of only a fifth of men who see their doctor with BOO symptoms.[22] However, two thirds are referred to a urologist, of whom four fifths are offered surgery, which nine out of ten accept. So only a fifth want an operation, but half end up having one (not necessarily including the fifth who initially wanted one). Urologists are not very good at telling men what having prostate surgery implies. The use of a leaflet detailing the advantages and disadvantages of trans-urethral resection of prostate (TURP) results in a quarter of men declining surgery, and another half having considerable reservations about it.[9]

TURP is offered as first choice by 90% of urologists.[22] Three quarters of those operated on are symptomatically improved.[23] It involves four or five days in hospital. Operative mortality is about 2%. One in seven patients gets a urinary infection, and one in eight loses enough blood to need transfusion.[24] In the longer term, retrograde ejaculation is about 100%.[11] One in eight end up incontinent, and one in five impotent (though one in ten get better erections after TURP).[24] One in five will need the operation re-doing within eight years because symptoms have returned.[22]

Open prostatectomy is more likely to be offered when the prostate is very big. An average of nine days in hospital is needed, and the chance of a urinary infection or significant bleed is greater than after TURP. In the longer term, about 1% of men become completely incontinent, and a third are impotent.[24]

Prostate cancer

Around 15 000 new cases of prostate cancer are notified each year in the UK.[2] Rates are very high in the US, and very low in Asia. Lifestyle may be important, as immigrants acquire the same risk of prostate cancer as the host population, but as yet there is no conclusive evidence to support lifestyle modification.[4]

Prostate cancer is usually very slowly progressive with a tumour size doubling time of around two years. About three quarters of prostate cancer sufferers are alive after one year and just under half at five years.[2] Overall only a minority – 39% – of men who contract prostate cancer will die because of it,[25] and in the elderly with the disease only 20% will die of their cancer and 80% will die of something unrelated.[2]

In the past a 'wait and see' policy has been advised, as there remains no conclusive evidence that the early treatment of prostate cancer prolongs life.[3] However, this is probably a reflection of the quality of the evidence, and seems implausible. Newer work suggests that treating prostate cancer adds an average of two years of life in the over 75s, and 14 years in the under 50s.[4] Treatment of prostate cancer now is no more likely to prolong life than it was in 1985.[2]

Localised prostate cancer is usually treated with *radical prostatectomy*, an open approach with removal of the prostate, its capsule, and the seminal vesicles. Even with nerve-sparing procedures, the rate of incontinence is high, and two thirds are completely impotent.[26] If bone metastases have occurred, then *androgen blockade* is a better option, with 80% of men having remission of bone pain for a median of 15 months. Survival is not increased, but quality of life is improved.[4] *Orchidectomy* has been used for 50 years or more. Gonadotrophin-releasing hormone (GnRH) analogues such as *gosorelin* are an option, and they also suppress the 5% of androgen which is made in the adrenals.

The median survival time after bone metastases have been diagnosed is 30 months.[3] Relapses eventually become resistant to hormone manipulation. *Local radiotherapy* can be useful palliation for bone pain, giving relief in 80% of instances.[3]

To screen or not?

The American Cancer Society recommends an annual PSA and DRE for all men over 40 years old. This may in part explain why radical prostatectomy for early prostate cancer is six times commoner in the US than in Britain.[26] British authorities disagree with screening routinely,[27] but suggest specifically looking for prostate cancer only in men with symptoms of BOO. Why has this divergence of opinion occurred?

- Prostate cancer may be genuinely *more prevalent* in the US. The sensitivity and specificity of a screening test will depend on the community prevalence of the disease being screened for. Screening may make sense in the US, but not over here
- The enthusiasm for screening in the US may reflect a more *general trend* towards medical intervention, encouraged by the high levels of health resources available for at least some sectors of US society
- Under half of men with diagnosed prostate cancer will die from it. If necropsy specimens are looked at, undiagnosed prostate cancer is about 10 times commoner than diagnosed prostate cancer. If all those cancers were detected premorbidly, 27 patients would be treated for only one who would have died of the disease.[12] This might not be considered a *sensible use of resources*, especially as treatment does not improve survival very much particularly in the older patient
- A combination of DRE, PSA and rectal ultrasound on one occasion will detect cancer in 2.5% of men.[11] Tumours under 5 mm are unlikely to be detected, but these are the ones which are also least likely to cause symptoms and mortality
- Educating patients about the advantages and disadvantages of PSA makes them less likely to want to be tested.[27] It is recommended that *before*

having a PSA test for screening purposes men need information[28] on the facts that

> The test can produce false-positive and false-negative results
> It is not known whether PSA screening reduces mortality
> The benefits of treating early prostate cancer are uncertain
> It is a blood test, and patients may worry about the results
> Prostate cancer is often incurable when symptoms appear
> Prostate cancer may not cause symptoms
> PSA can detect cancer earlier than DRE
> PSA screening is controversial.

Using a DRE and PSA of over 3 ng/ml, a reduction in prostate cancer deaths of 70% has been reported.[29] Based on these figures, it is cheaper to prevent a prostate cancer death than it is to prevent one from breast or cervical cancer.

- Symptoms of bladder outflow obstruction are very common in elderly men, and half of symptoms are not reported to a doctor
- Basic examination and investigations for a man with symptoms consists of: abdominal and rectal examination; MSU and blood for PSA and U&E
- Not all men want treatment for their symptoms, and a few will get better untreated
- Medications available for BPH will help over half of men, but all can affect sexual functioning
- Most men referred to a urologist with symptoms of bladder outflow obstruction will get an operation
- Screening for prostate cancer is not recommended in the United Kingdom, but is recommended in the USA.

💬 Topics for discussion

- Incontinence is a filthy habit that lazy old men sometimes get themselves into
- All men get prostate cancer if they live long enough. It isn't worth worrying about
- Prostate surgery is six times commoner in the US than in Britain. Why?
- Men should get a PSA and a DRE if they ask for it.

📖 References

1. Muir G. Benign prostatic disease. *General Practitioner* February 13, 1998: 58–60.
2. Kirby M. Incidence of prostate cancer continues to rise. *Medical Monitor* 11 October 2000: 43–4.
3. Dearnaley D P. Cancer of the prostate. *BMJ* 1994; 308: 780–4.
4. Muir G. Prostate cancer. *General Practitioner* May 1 1998: 60–62.
5. Simpson R J. Benign prostatic hyperplasia. *Br J Gen Pract* 1997; 47: 235–40.
6. Hunter D J W, McKee C M, Black N A et al. Urinary symptoms: prevalence and severity in British men. *J Epidemiol Comm Health* 1994; 48: 569–75.

7. Cunningham-Burley S, Allbutt H, Garraway W M et al. Perceptions of urinary symptoms and health-care-seeking behaviour amongst men aged 40–79 years. *Br J Gen Pract* 1996; 46: 349–52.
8. Thomas T, Plymat K, Blannin J et al. Prevalence of urinary incontinence. *BMJ* 1980; 281: 1243–5.
9. Hunter D J W, McKee C M, Black N A et al. Health care sought and received by men with urinary symptoms and their views on prostatectomy. *Br J Gen Pract* 1995; 45: 27–30.
10. Farmer A. *10 Minute consultation:* Prostatic symptoms. *BMJ* 2001; 322: 1468.
11. Williams G. Prostatic problems. *Care of the Elderly* 1993; 5: 265–8.
12. Scroder F H. Prostate cancer: to screen or not to screen? *BMJ* 1993; 306: 407–8.
13. Clarke N W. Prostate cancer. *Update* 1992; 47: 605–14.
14. Dawson C and Whitfield H. ABC of urology: bladder outflow obstruction. *BMJ* 1996; 312: 767–70.
15. Simak R, Madersbacher S, Zhang Z F et al. The impact of ejaculation on serum prostate specific antigen. *J Urol* 1993; 150: 895–7.
16. PSA and screening. *Bandolier* 1996; 3: 7.
17. Payne S. Current management of prostatic problems. *Update* 1996; 52: 184–92.
18. Simpson R J, Lee R J, Garraway W M et al. Consultation patterns in a community survey of men with benign prostatic hyperplasia. *Br J Gen Pract* 1994; 44: 499–502.
19. MacPherson S. How to shrink a prostate. *General Practitioner* March 4, 1994: 29.
20. Wein A J. Evaluation of treatment response to drugs in benign prostatic hyperplasia. *Urol Clin N Am* 1990; 17: 631–40.
21. British National Formulary 41 (March 2001). London: BMA/RPSGB, 2001.
22. Shreeve C. Benign prostatic hypertrophy. *The Practitioner* 1993; 237: 619–23.
23. Bruskewitz R C, Larsen E H, Madson P O et al. Three year follow-up of urinary symptoms after transurethral resection of the prostate. *J Urol* 1986; 136: 613–5.
24. Nuffield Institute for Health, University of Leeds; NHS Centre for Reviews and Dissemination, University of York. Effective Health Care: *Benign Prostatic Hyperplasia* 1995; 2(2).
25. Minerva. *BMJ* 2000; 320: 1416.
26. Minerva. *BMJ* 1997; 315: 556.
27. Woolf S H. Should we screen for prostate cancer? *BMJ* 1997; 314: 989–90.
28. Chan E C and Sulmasy D P. What men should know about prostate-specific antigen screening before giving informed consent. *Am J Med* 1998; 105(4): 266–74.
29. Charatan F B. Prostate cancer screening reduces deaths. *BMJ* 1998; 316: 1626.

Breast problems

Tutorial aim **The registrar can appropriately assess and manage breast problems in primary care.**

Learning objectives By the end of the tutorial the registrar can:

- Take an appropriate breast history
- Clinically examine a female breast
- Manage mastalgia
- Deal with nipple discharge
- Appropriately manage breast lumps
- Discuss with a patient the treatment of breast cancer
- Plan a programme of psychological support for a patient with breast cancer
- Counsel a woman about breast cancer screening.

Introduction

In a given year around 3% of all women experience breast problems sufficiently troublesome to consult their GP.[1] Each year in the UK over 30 000 new breast cancers are diagnosed, and 14 000 women die of the disease.[2] Breast cancer is the leading cause of cancer death in women aged 40 to 50,[3] and the commonest single cause of all deaths in women aged 35 to 54.[4] Comparing this with other important cancers in women, there are each year about 4500 cases and 2200 deaths from cancer of the cervix, 5000 cases and 4300 deaths from cancer of the ovary, and 3750 cases and 1000 deaths from cancer of the uterus.[5]

Breast cysts affect 7% of all women.[6]

Three quarters of all women experience breast pain.[7] In most cases it is of mild or moderate severity.

Breast lumps

Most breast lumps are not due to cancer, especially in younger women. However, when a lump is found the prospect of cancer will be uppermost in the woman's mind. Much of the management of breast lumps is directed towards the detection or exclusion of cancer.

Benign breast lumps

These can be of three types:

- Fibroadenoma

- Cyst
- Nodularity.

The chance of finding each type of benign lump varies with the age of the woman. The chance of a lump being cancerous also varies with age: in women under 44 years, only 3% of lumps are cancer, but in women aged 55 (postmenopausal) the risk is 48%.[4] Lumps are commoner in younger women, but are less likely to be cancer.

Fibroadenomas are smooth, rounded and up to 5 cm across. When palpated they will often slip from the grasp, leading to their other name of *breast mouse*. They are much commoner in younger women and are present in 60% of 20-year-olds, but only 5% of 50-year-olds:[6] they account for 13% of all breast lumps found.

The chance of a *breast cyst* is maximum at age 50 with 30% of all women affected. Cysts account for 15% of all discrete breast masses.[6] Diagnosis is established by fine needle aspiration. Between 1% and 3% of women with cysts also have a carcinoma.

The peak age for *nodularity* is 30 years, with 60% of all women being affected. There is a wide age range, however, and this is the commonest reason for a breast mass, with 38% of all breast masses turning out to be due to nodularity. Against a background of lumpiness there are often areas of fibrosis or sclerosis which present as lumps. This was previously termed *mastitis*.

Taking a breast history

Important questions include

- How long has the lump been present?
- Is it changing? Is it growing?
- Does it alter with the menstrual cycle?
- Are there any associated symptoms?
- Is there any personal or family history which might be relevant?

The risk of breast cancer varies with

- *Age* The most important risk factor. Breast cancer is rare under age 30, and the incidence roughly doubles with each decade thereafter until the menopause, when the rate of increase slows appreciably.[8] Eighty per cent of all new breast cancer diagnoses and 88% of deaths occur in the over-50 age group.[4]
- *Family History* About 5% of breast cancers are linked to specific single gene defects. Carriers of the BRCA1 mutation have a lifetime risk of 80% for breast cancer and 20–40% for ovarian cancer.[9] Identifying the carriers of such genes is difficult.

📄 **Guidelines**   **Significant family history in breast cancer[10]**

The risk of breast cancer quadruples in women who have

Four or more relatives with breast or ovarian cancer
Three relatives of median age under 60 with ovarian or breast cancer
Two relatives of median age under 40 with breast cancer
Any relative with both breast and ovarian cancer.

- *Gender* About 0.5% of all breast cancers occur in men. The peak incidence is about 10 years later than in women. The histology and prognosis for each tumour stage is the same as for women.[11]
- *Late first pregnancy* Women who have a first full-term pregnancy after the age of 35 carry three times the risk of women who are first pregnant below age 20.[12]
- *Early menarche* Women who begin menstruating at age 10 have three times the breast cancer risk of those who begin at age 15.[12]
- *Late menopause* Women whose periods stop at 55 have twice the breast cancer risk of those who stop aged 45.[8]
- *Previous breast cancer.*

Breast examination

There are a number of ways to examine breasts. Whichever is chosen, it is important to be consistent and careful. Examination is best done in the first two weeks of the menstrual cycle.

- Ask the woman to undress to the waist and then sit upright with the arms down. Observe the breast contours
- Ask the woman to lift her arms above her head, and observe again
- Ask the woman to lie down on a couch with its head raised at 30°, arms by her sides
- Start by examining the asymptomatic breast
- Using the flat of the hand or straight fingers, palpate the breast against the chest wall. Either start at the nipple and work outwards in a spiral, or palpate the four quadrants in turn
- Feel for axillary lumps
- Ask the woman to sit leaning slightly forward, and palpate the breasts again.

Clinical features suggesting a malignant lesion are:

- *A discrete lump.* About three quarters present in this way.[13] Around 90% of breast cancers are found by the women themselves or their partners.[4] Hard craggy lumps which are growing and do not alter with the menstrual cycle are particularly suspicious
- *Tethering.* A cancerous breast lump may be fixed to the chest wall or to the overlying skin, causing it to pucker. The nipple may recently have become retracted

- *Axillary Mass.* Malignant regional lymph nodes are hard, matted and may be fixed to underlying structures
- *Other features.* The presence of *peau d'orange* indicates that there is inflammation present with a corresponding poor prognosis. *Paget's disease* of the nipple is found in only 2% of all breast cancers, but in this group 75% will prove to have invasive carcinoma.[11] More rarely there may be *swelling* of the breast, pain or nipple *discharge*.

Guidelines   Referring breast lumps[1]

A woman with a breast lump should be referred to a specialist when

- A discrete lump is found on clinical examination
- There is asymmetrical nodularity, patient over 35
- There is asymmetrical nodularity, patient under 35 with strong family history
- There is asymmetrical nodularity, patient under 35 with no family history, but clinical findings persist after review at six weeks.

Breast pain

Types of breast pain

Distinguishing the three types of breast pain requires clinical examination and information about how the pain fits with the menstrual cycle. A *menstrual diary* may help.

Cyclical mastalgia occurs in 65% of cases and the pain varies with the menstrual cycle.[7] The average age of sufferers is 34. Normally many women experience a heightened awareness, discomfort, fullness and heaviness of the breasts during the three to seven days before menses. In cyclical mastalgia there is increasingly severe pain from about mid cycle. The breasts feel heavy and are tender to touch. Typically the outer parts of the breasts are more severely affected, and pain is more severe after physical activity, especially lifting. The pain may fluctuate in severity from cycle to cycle, and can persist for years. The menopause always relieves the symptoms, but pregnancy, the oral contraceptive pill and parity do not.[7]

In *non-cyclical mastalgia* the typical sufferer is aged 43. Pain may fluctuate in severity, but not with the menstrual cycle. Pain is often localised and described as 'burning' or 'drawing' in character.

In some women the pain does not originate in the breasts at all, but from the *chest wall*. Tender spots may be palpable either on the intercostal muscles, or the costo-chondral junctions (the aptly named *Teitze's disease*). There may be a history of minor trauma or aches and strains: once the pain has started the muscle tension produced by anxiety over the implication of the symptom prolongs the clinical course. There may be a parallel with the fit young man with chest pain who fears serious heart disease. It is hard to rest damaged intercostal muscles, unless you can persuade the sufferer to hold their breath for a fortnight.

Managing breast pain

📄 **Guidelines**

Treating breast pain[1]

Examine the breasts to exclude a discrete mass. Breast cancer can cause pain. If there is

- Mild to moderate cyclical mastalgia   Explain nature of problem
- Severe cyclical mastalgia (15%)   First line is to offer gamolenic acid
- Mild to moderate non-cyclical mastalgia   Second line danazol or bromocriptine
- Severe non-cyclical mastalgia   Explain nature of problem
  If localized, REFER
  If diffuse offer gamolenic acid,
  danazol or bromocriptine

With *reassurance* and a normal clinical examination, up to 85% of women will not wish further treatment of their pain.[7] A well-fitted bra worn at night can ease symptoms appreciably. In the treatment of breast pain, a placebo effect of 19% has been found.[14]

Women with breast pain have no more psychiatric morbidity than the general population.[7] Mastalgia is not a psychiatric disorder in spite of what is written is some of the older textbooks, usually by male gynaecologists.

Gamolenic acid, six to eight 40 mg capsules a day (in two doses), will help 38% of women with cyclical or non-cyclical mastalgia.[7] The maximum effects may not be achieved until after four months of treatment.[14] Side effects are mild (nausea) and affect only 2% of users.[15] Though expensive this is probably the treatment of first choice.

Danazol, 100 mg to 300 mg a day, will help 79% of women with cyclical mastalgia and 40% of women with non-cyclical mastalgia: but 30% will have side effects (weight gain, acne, hirsutism).[7] Treatment may take two months to achieve benefit.

Bromocriptine, 2.5 mg a day helps 54% of women with cyclical and 35% of women with non-cyclical mastalgia.[7] However unwanted effects (nausea, headache, postural hypotension and constipation) occur in 33% of users and are severe in 15%.[14]

For *chest wall pain*, explanation and reassurance can be used in generous measure. Non-steroidal anti-inflammatory medications are also worth a try. If a localised spot of tenderness can be found, an injection of local anaesthetic and steroid will help in up to 60% of cases.[7]

📄 **Guidelines**

Managing nipple discharge[1]

Lump present   manage as for lump

No lump present and patient is under 50
multiple ducts involved, or discharge bloodstained   REFER

single duct	REFER
large volume	REFER
small volume, clear or coloured	explain
No lump, patient is over 50	REFER

Breast cancer

- Each woman in the UK has a lifetime risk of 1 in 12 of contracting breast cancer.[16] The UK has the highest mortality from breast cancer in the world, accounting for 18% of all cancers in women[8] and 20% of all cancer deaths[5]
- The number of breast cancer sufferers is rising throughout the world[3]
- After five years, 62% of breast cancer sufferers are alive, compared with 58% for cancer of the cervix, 28% for cancer of the ovary and 70% for cancer of the uterus[17]
- The prognosis for advanced breast cancer has altered little in the last 30 years, but the outlook for sufferers from early breast cancer has got better.[15] Overall, in the UK the prognosis for breast cancer is slowly improving,[18] and the death rate is declining.[9]

Diagnosis

Breast pathology is very common, and women are rightly concerned if a lump is found. Only a minority of lumps found by self-examination will turn out to be malignant, especially in younger women.

A more complete diagnosis of a breast lump can only be made by *triple assessment* at a specialist centre,[3] involving clinical examination, fine needle aspiration cytology (FNAC) and diagnostic mammography. The clinical examination will be broadly a repeat of the examination already performed, but done by a doctor with a special interest and expertise in breast lumps.

FNAC involves the insertion of a needle, usually of 'green barrel' gauge, into the lump, sometimes under mammographic guidance. This will determine whether the lump is solid or not, and may yield fluid for histological analysis. An anaesthetic is not usually required. Some specialists are so confident in their technique that unless the fluid is bloodstained it is not sent for cytological analysis, and if any cyst can be aspirated to extinction then the woman is discharged from further follow up.[3]

Diagnostic mammography involves a number of views, and not the single oblique view currently used for screening mammography. About 18% of palpable breast cancers will yield a normal mammogram,[3] and so it is important that this is not the only basis of the diagnosis and that a full assessment is made.

The government decided that from 1 April 1999 all cases of suspected breast cancer would be seen in a specialist clinic within two weeks of referral. Delays may possibly worsen the eventual prognosis, and they certainly worsen the psychological burden on the woman. Units with an interest in breast cancer generally achieve better results from treatment, a topic which has recently stimulated the Cancer Relief Macmillan Fund to campaign for minimum standards to be applied to units treating breast cancer.[19] Such a unit should be available and within reach of all patients in the UK.

Mortality

Over half of women with breast cancer survive to die of something else. Breast cancer accounts for 4% of all female deaths, whereas coronary heart disease is responsible for 43%.[20] A woman smoker over 50 is more likely to die from lung cancer than from breast cancer.[21]

📁 **Evidence**

> **Staging breast cancer survival[22]**
>
> Using the International Union Against Cancer stages, the mortality from breast cancer is:
>
> - Stage I : localised lump with no nodes involved. Five year survival 90%
> - Stage II: localised lump with nodes involved. Five year survival 60%
> - Stage III: locally advanced disease, clinical evidence of infiltration of the skin or chest wall, or matted axillary lymph nodes. Five year survival 40%
> - Stage IV: distant metastases present. Five year survival 10%.

Four fifths of breast cancers present at the stage where they are technically resectable, and these have the best prognosis.[23] In fact, in about half of these cases it will be apparent by the clinical course of the disease that the lymph nodes were already involved at the time of diagnosis.[3] However this does not materially affect management or outcome.

Surgery

For cancers up to 2 cm across, and possibly for cancers up to 5 cm, *mastectomy* and *conservation surgery with radiotherapy* carry equal chances of survival.[24] Mastectomy is a bigger and more mutilating operation. Conservation surgery consists either of removing the lump with a tumour-free margin (the so-called *lumpectomy*), or else removing the breast quadrant containing the tumour. Both these are combined with either axillary clearance or sampling. Not all tumours can be treated with conservation surgery. Those over 4 cm usually require a mastectomy. However, it is sometimes possible to shrink a tumour down to 4 cm using chemotherapy so that breast conservation can be achieved.[23] In up to 80% of cases of large localised breast tumour, and 25% of locally advanced disease, the tumour mass can be shrunk by systemic therapy to a point where breast conservation surgery is possible.[25]

Local tumour recurrence is greater after conservation surgery at between 5% and 21%.[3] This does not, however, affect the death rate from the disease. It is straightforward to perform a mastectomy after initial conservation surgery.

The *psychological consequences* of mastectomy and conservation surgery are about the same, with 35% to 40% of women suffering anxiety, depression or both in the two years following either procedure.[15] Though preservation of the breast has important benefits in terms of self image, it may lead to women being less secure in the belief that the cancer has gone, causing obsessive concern over breast symptoms.

The best way to secure psychological health after breast cancer surgery is to involve the woman fully in management decisions. There is some evidence that this is being achieved to a greater extent than in the past.[19] While it is good practice to encourage breast cancer sufferers to choose their preferred treatment, doing so also means that it will in future not be possible to do randomised trials comparing mastectomy and conservation surgery.

The cosmetic results after mastectomy tend to improve with time. After conservation surgery the opposite is often the case because of the longer-term effects of radiotherapy.[3] Breast reconstruction is done in about 10% of women after mastectomy,[26] whereas about 50% would like it. Any problems following the surgery will depend on the particular technique used. Reconstruction does not, however, lead to an increased chance of tumour recurrence.[26]

Adjuvant treatment

Radiotherapy

In women treated with lumpectomy and axillary node dissection, recurrence rates are less if subsequent radiotherapy is used.[15] Treatment is to the tumour bed in all cases, and also to the axilla if the nodes have been sampled rather than cleared. Radiotherapy and axillary clearance together is avoided as this invariably leads to *lymphoedema* of the arm. Around 30 treatments are needed over several weeks or months. This will involve repeated visits to the treatment centre. Other problems are that the cosmetic result of surgery tends to be worse because of *radiation scarring*, and there is an increased incidence of ischaemic heart disease.[3] Larger more focused doses of radiation can be achieved by implants.

Chemotherapy

Chemotherapy improves the outlook particularly in advanced breast cancer.[16] Death from the disease is not avoided, but life can be prolonged. In early breast cancer, chemotherapy improves survival by 16% and recurrence by 28%,[15] with benefit being greatest for women under 50 years. However the survival rate in early breast cancer patients is very good anyway, and so even an impressive relative improvement in mortality of about a sixth does not represent much in terms of women alive who would otherwise be dead. The benefits of chemotherapy have to be balanced against the disadvantages. Six treatments are usually needed.[15] The commonest side effects of treatment are tiredness, nausea, loss of appetite, mouth soreness, pain, sickness and sore eyes. Each patient will get between five and seven side effects.[27]

Endocrine therapy

Ovarian ablation in the under-50 age group reduces recurrence by 26% and improves survival by 25% in early breast cancer.[15] There is an additive effect with chemotherapy.

Tamoxifen is primarily an anti-oestrogen, but in some respects has oestrogenic properties. Its use improves survival by 17% and recurrence by 25%. It also reduces the chance of recurrence in the other breast by 39%.[15] Women over 50 do better with tamoxifen, as do those with oestrogen receptor-positive tumours. However some benefit is seen in all tumour types. Treatment is known to be effective for up to two years, and benefits may be seen up to five years. It is usually well tolerated though hot flushes, vaginal bleeding and gastro-intestinal symptoms can be caused. Its oestrogen agonist properties prevent tamoxifen causing osteoporosis and ischaemic heart disease.

Psychological support for breast cancer sufferers

The rate of anxiety and depression in women diagnosed as having breast cancer in the previous year is about four times that of the general population.[28] Most units now have trained counsellors or *mastectomy nurses* who have often had breast cancer treatment themselves. Early involvement is useful to discuss the nature and implications of treatments. While there is little evidence that such counselling prevents psychological morbidity, the identification of 'at risk' patients is helpful. The use of a psychiatrist or psychologist will reduce the rate of psychological morbidity by 75%.[28]

After or during treatment, a loss reaction is apparent. This reaction has many of the characteristics of a bereavement reaction, modified because the female breast serves a wide variety of social and sexual functions. Problems with body image after mastectomy are especially common (20 to 30%) and these patients are more likely to develop anxiety or a depressive disorder. Advice about implants and clothing may be useful.

Up to a quarter of women who undergo chemotherapy develop a *conditioned response*: any stimulus which reminds them of the treatment causes a re-emergence of the side affects of treatment such as nausea and vomiting.[28]

Further support and information can be obtained from self-help organisations:

Self-help groups

Breast Care and Mastectomy Association of Great Britain
15-19 Britten Street
London SW3 3TZ
020 7867 1103

British Association of Cancer United Patients (BACUP)
Freeline 0800 181 199
or Information Line 020 7613 2121

Preventing breast cancer

Mammography

Breast screening by mammography was the first cancer screening method demonstrated to be of value in rigorous randomised trials.[29] Screening mammography is a low intensity X-ray technique which can detect cancers 1 cm or less across. It is not particularly pleasant, with 81% of women experiencing discomfort. This is classified as actual pain by 46% of women, and 7% describe the pain as severe.[4]

As long as target levels can be achieved for population coverage, the research suggests that over a 12-year period a mammography screening programme will reduce breast cancer mortality by 29% overall and by 40% in those who attend for screening.[29] Figures from the NHS Mammography Programme up to 1998 showed a 21.3% reduction in breast cancer mortality, but only 6.4% of this was attributed to mammography while 14.9% was attributed to better treatment.[30] The breast cancers detected by mammography are more likely to be at an early stage than those detected by other methods, so that in 70 to 80% a good prognosis can be expected.[4]

Following the recommendations of the Forrest Report (1986),[31] the UK Mammography Programme was set up in 1988 just before a general election. Women aged from 50 to 64 are invited for a mammogram every three years, with continuation thereafter at the request of the woman. From late 2001 the scheme is to be extended to invite all women up to age 74.[9] Using the UK screening methods benefit is only seen in the over-50 age group. Mammography of the premenopausal breast is less likely to pick up clinically useful information,[4] partly because the breast tissue is more dense and partly because premenopausal breast cancer often follows a slightly different clinical course.

The effectiveness of the mammography programme is limited, particularly in the early years, by a number of factors.[32]

- The *sensitivity* of screening mammography is only around 95%
- *Lead time bias*: in the early stages of the programme, some breast cancers which have been present for a long time may be found. Mortality from cases of more advanced breast cancer is a lot higher
- *Length bias sampling*: some cancers are detected which are so slow growing that they would not cause problems during the lifetime of the patient.

In order for a mammography programme to produce a significant reduction in mortality an attendance for screening rate of over 70% must be achieved.[29] The acceptance rate for 1998/99 was 75.5%.[33]

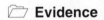 **Evidence**

GP implications of mammography:[29,34]

Based on a GP list of 2000:

- 150 women will be eligible for screening
- 113 will attend for screening
- 8 will get recalled for further investigation
- 1 or 2 will have a biopsy
- under 1 will have cancer.

For each cancer found, around 11 other women will be unnecessarily worried.

Further concern is caused by the rate of *interval cancer* being found, that is breast cancers which arise between mammograms. Two-view mammography increases the detection of breast cancers by 20%, and there is a further 15% increase if two radiologists read the films.[35] Since in some studies internationally the rate of interval cancer is nearly as high as the rate of detected cancer,[36] such an improved detection rate is very important. Two-view screening mammography would be cost effective.[37] The chance of interval cancer is highest in the third year after mammography. Under a recent change, the UK programme now offers two views on the first screening.[33]

Examination

It is logical to expect an improvement in breast cancer prognosis in women who regularly examine their own breasts and report any lumps found. Women who practise breast self-examination (BSE) are more likely to find lumps less than 2 cm across and are less likely to have axillary deposits at diagnosis.[38] In population studies, however, BSE has not been shown to reduce the death rate from breast cancer. Research in this area is limited by a lack of consensus about what a BSE should consist of and how frequently it should be done.[4] Arbitrarily a monthly examination following menses is usually advised.

The government's advice to women now is not that they should BSE regularly, but that they should be *breast aware*, and report any perceived changes to their GP.[39] Breast awareness is achieved by[4]

- Knowing what is normal for you
- Looking and feeling
- Knowing what changes to look out for:

  change in the outline, shape or size
  puckering or dimpling of the skin
  any discrete new lump
  persistent asymmetrical nodularity early in cycle
  pain or discomfort which is different from normal for you
  recent onset nipple discharge, especially if bloody
  persistent single duct discharge
  nipple retraction or distortion

- Reporting any changes without delay
- Attending for breast screening when invited.

Recent work has suggested that breast examination by a nurse or doctor is as effective as mammography in reducing breast cancer mortality. Mammography detects smaller cancers, but over 13 years this does not influence mortality.[40] Further evidence is awaited.

Summary

- Breast problems are very common in general practice. For example, most women will have breast pain at some time in their life
- Most breast lumps are not malignant, especially in women under 35
- Under government guidance, suspected breast cancer has to be seen by a specialist within two weeks of referral
- Mammography probably reduces breast cancer mortality, but routine breast self-examination does not
- Clear guidelines have been published for the management of breast problems
- Treatment for breast cancer is prolonged and unpleasant, and carries physical and psychological morbidity.

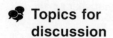 Topics for discussion

- In pre-menopausal women, discrete breast lumps can safely be left to see if they resolve after the next menses

- The key to future breast cancer mortality reduction is the development of new treatments
- All women should be offered breast reconstruction after a mastectomy
- Breast pain is a normal part of being a woman
- Male doctors should insist on a female chaperone being present when performing breast examination
- Should GPs aspirate breast cysts?

📖 References

1. Austoker J and Mansel R. Guidelines for referral of patients with breast problems. Sheffield: NHS Breast Screening Programme, 1999.
2. Jones J. Breast cancer treatment delays affect survival. *BMJ* 1999; 318: 959.
3. Benson J R, Lau Y, Jatoi I et al. Early breast cancer: diagnosis and management. *Update* 1993; 47: 337–44.
4. Austoker J. Screening and self examination for breast cancer. *BMJ* 1994; 309: 168–74.
5. Austoker J and Sharp D. Breast screening: a subject for debate. *Br J Gen Pract* 1991; 41: 166–7.
6. Dixon J M and Mansel R E. ABC of Breast Diseases: Congenital problems and aberrations of normal breast development and involution. *BMJ* 1994; 309: 797–800.
7. Mansel R E. ABC of Breast Diseases: Breast pain. *BMJ* 1994, 309: 866–8.
8. McPherson K, Steel C M and Dixon J M. *ABC of breast diseases:* Breast cancer – epidemiology, risk factors, and genetics. *BMJ* 2000; 321: 624–8.
9. Jone A. Breast cancer – part one. *General Practitioner* January 26 2001, 34–5.
10. British Association of Surgical Oncology Guidelines. *Eur J Surg Oncol* 1998; 244: 64–76.
11. Dixon J M, Sainsbury J R C and Rodger A. Breast cancer: treatment of elderly patients and uncommon conditions. *BMJ* 1994; 309: 1292–5.
12. Evans D G R, Fentiman I S, McPherson K et al. Familial breast cancer. *BMJ* 1994; 308: 183–7.
13. The Yorkshire Breast Cancer Group. Symptoms and signs of operable breast cancer. *Br J Surg* 1983; 70: 350–2.
14. Cyclical breast pain – what works and what doesn't. *Drug and Therapeutics Bulletin* 1992; 30: 1–3.
15. Management of early breast cancer. *Drug and Therapeutics Bulletin* 1992; 30: 53–6.
16. Jones A L and Smith I E. Medical treatment of breast cancer. *Update* 1993; 47: 505–12.
17. Austoker J. Cancer prevention: setting the scene. *BMJ* 1994; 308: 1415–20.
18. Brown P. UK death rates from breast cancer fall by a third. *BMJ* 2000; 321: 849.
19. Cancer charity boosts patients' expectations. *General Practitioner* May 20 1994.
20. Drew S. What is the true risk of breast cancer? *Update* 1999; 58: 1006–7.
21. Bunker J P, Houghton J and Baum M. Putting the risk of breast cancer in perspective. *BMJ* 1998; 317: 1307–9.
22. Sainsbury J R C, Anderson T J and Morgan D A L. *ABC of breast diseases:* Breast cancer. *BMJ* 2000; 321: 745–50.
23. Rubens R D. Management of early breast cancer. *BMJ* 1992; 304: 1361–4.
24. Gottleib S. Lumpectomy as good as mastectomy for tumours up to 5 cm. *BMJ* 2000; 32: 261.
25. Dixon M J. Surgery and radiotherapy for early breast cancer. *BMJ* 1995; 311: 1515–16.

26. O'Donnell M. Reconstructive surgery after mastectomy. *The Practitioner* 1994; 238: 261–5.
27. Tierney A J, Leonard R C F, Taylor J et al. Side effects expected and experienced by women receiving chemotherapy for breast cancer. *BMJ* 1991; 302: 272.
28. Maguire P. ABC of Breast Diseases: psychological aspects. *BMJ* 1994; 309: 1649–52.
29. Blamey R W, Wilson A R M and Patnick J. *ABC of breast diseases:* Screening for breast cancer. *BMJ* 2000; 321: 689–93.
30. Blanks R G, Moss S M, McGahan C E *et al.* Effect of NHS breast screening programme on mortality from breast cancer in England and Wales, 1990–8: comparison of observed with predicted mortality. *BMJ* 2000; 321: 665–9.
31. Forrest P. Breast cancer screening. London: HMSO, 1986.
32. Michell M J. Breast screening. *Update* 1992; 43: 954–8.
33. Ferriman A. Detection rates for breast cancer rising. *BMJ* 2000; 321: 1101.
34. Austoker J. Breast cancer screening and the primary care team. *BMJ* 1990; 300: 1631–4.
35. Field S, Michell M J, Wallis M G W et al. What should be done about interval breast cancers? *BMJ* 1995; 310: 203–4.
36. Van Dijck J A A M, Verbeek A L M, Hendrix J H C L et al. The current detectability of breast cancer in a mammographic screening program. *Cancer* 1993; 72: 1933–8.
37. Wald J W, Murphy P, Major P et al. UKCCCR multicentre randomised controlled trial of one and two view mammography in breast cancer screening. *BMJ* 1995; 311: 1189–93.
38. Fentiman I S. Recent developments in the surgical treatment of breast cancer. *Maternal and Child Health,* 1992; 17: 185–90.
39. Calman K C and Poole A A B. PL/CMO(91)15 29th November 1991 Department of Health, London.
40. Mittra I, Baum M, Thornton H and Houghton J. Is clinical breast examination an acceptable alternative to mammographic screening? *BMJ* 2000; 321: 1071–3.

Child abuse

Tutorial aim	**The registrar is aware of presentations which might indicate child abuse, and can use an appropriate child abuse procedure.**
Learning objectives	By the end of the tutorial the registrar can: <ul><li>List five presentations suggestive of child physical abuse</li><li>List five presentations suggestive of child sexual abuse</li><li>Discuss the requirements of a consultation for child abuse with respect to history-taking, examination, and record-keeping</li><li>Decide how and when to take advice in possible child abuse</li><li>Discuss the GP's role in child abuse proceedings</li><li>Take an appropriately professional view of the ongoing care of an abusing family.</li></ul>

Some background

In March 1995 there were about 35 000 children on child protection registers in England,[1] a rate of about 3.5 per 1000 children under age 18.[2] However, the incidence of violence against children is much higher than this. According to the National Commission on the Prevention of Child Abuse (1996), child abuse is '*Anything which individuals, institutions, or processes do or fail to do which directly or indirectly harms children or damages their prospects of safe and healthy development into adulthood*'. Using such a definition, up to one million children are abused each year.[1] This includes:

- 150 000 who are physically harmed
- 100 000 who have potentially harmful sexual experiences
- 400 000 who lack a caring environment
- 250 000 who witness violence among parents or carers.

Most abused children do not end up on a child protection register. Each GP will on average have about 30 instances of child abuse among patients each year, but only one child on a protection register.

📁 **Evidence**

Categories of child abuse[1,3]	
• *Neglect*	32%
• *Physical injury*	37%
• *Sexual abuse*	26%
• *Emotional abuse*	13%
(9% in more than one category).	

Before the Children Act 1989, there was a further category of *Grave concern* which has now been discontinued. Under the old categories about a third of registrations were for *Grave concern*.[2]

Non-accidental injury (NAI) is a term covering all types of child abuse. Child sexual abuse (CSA) is considered separately.

Physical injury

A definition

Actual or likely physical injury to a child, or failure to prevent physical injury (or suffering) to a child including deliberate poisoning, suffocation and Munchausen's syndrome by proxy[2]

The term *battered baby syndrome* was coined by Kempe in the US in 1962. The existence of child abuse had been known for some time, but had been generally tolerated. In 1880 Lord Shaftesbury, fresh from his success in improving conditions for children at work, was nonetheless reluctant to do anything to protect children at home. At the time he was quoted as saying that legislation protecting children in the home *'Would not, I think, be entertained in either House of Parliament'*.[2]

A third of children in 'ordinary' two-parent families in Britain have been subject to severe physical punishment with the use, for example, of whips, canes, riding crops, electric flexes and belts.[4] The beating of children at school in Britain has in only the recent past been banned, and then only because such a ban was needed to comply with a European Court ruling. In a number of social groups, including some ethnic minorities, the physical punishment of children continues to be regarded as a necessary part of parenthood.

The victims of physical abuse

Boys and girls are both abused. Firstborn children are more often affected, and within a family it is common for just one of the children to be abused. Young children are most at risk, partly because they are more vulnerable to injury, and partly because they cannot seek help elsewhere. Children under two years are at greatest risk.

Severe physical abuse has a prevalence of one per 1000 in children under four years. Death from abuse is rare after the age of one, but there is a minimum mortality of one in 10 000 children, or about 100 per year in the UK.[2] In many cases the abuse occurs as the result of an angry outburst from the abuser. In a minority of cases the child is subjected to repeated and systematic abuse over a long period of time.

Abusing families

Most abuse is committed by the child's parents or those with parental responsibility, and it is particularly common for a carer or a cohabitee who is living in the home but not related to the child to be the abuser. Young parents are more likely to abuse than older ones. Abusing parents do not usually have an identified mental illness, though they may show *personality traits* predisposing to violent behaviour. They may be unable to provide appropriate care for or control of their children. Where a psychiatric disorder is present, it is most likely to be a puerperal or other type of *psychosis. Victims of drug or alcohol abuse* are more likely to abuse their children, as are parents under *stress* because of illness, bereavement or financial worries.[5] Child abuse is more common in the *socially deprived* and in families without employment, but it occurs in all strata of society.

People who abuse children are also statistically more likely to be *unwilling to wait* their turn to see the GP.[5] The GP who wishes to secure the safety of an abused child must be aware of this and respond promptly even if it means disrupting a surgery or an inappropriate use of the emergency services.

Abuse is calculated to be twenty times more likely if the parents were abused as children. On the other hand more than a third of mothers who were abused as children provide good care for their own children and do not abuse them.[2]

A priority for the GP must be to recognise the possibility that abuse has occurred, even if the family does not fit into the stereotype.

Detecting physical abuse

Pointers which should alert a GP that abuse may have occurred include:

- Delay in seeking advice and treatment for an injury
- The reported *circumstances* of the injury not matching the observed facts
- Injuries in young children not matching what is possible bearing in mind the child's developmental maturity. For example, children under one rarely hurt themselves by running into things as they are usually unable to run
- Abnormal interaction between child and parent. The child may be anxious or distant and the parent may ignore the child's behaviour or distress. There may be known child-rearing problems, sleeping or feeding difficulties
- An older child saying something which gives a clue to the diagnosis
- Multiple small injuries in young children
- *Disabled* children are at extra risk of abuse.

Presentations suspicious of physical abuse

Br uises

May be of different ages. They may occur on the face and round the mouth, and be caused by fingertips. There may be grip marks on the shoulders. Petechial haemorrhages can be associated with shaking, suffocation or strangling. Bruises to ears are unusual if not deliberately inflicted: the area is protected by the top of the skull and the shoulder tip, the *triangle of safety*. On the other hand, if examined, 12% of all babies have bruises, especially if the baby is mobile. These *normal bruises* are invariably on the front of the body, affecting particularly the head and other bony prominences.[6]

Scratches

Deliberately inflicted are usually *multiple and linear*. The edges of hard objects inflict linear marks. All bite marks need careful examination as they readily become infected.

Mouth injuries

May be caused by blows to the mouth, or by forcing things into the mouth. A *ruptured frenulum* is a typical injury.

Fractures

May be *multiple and of different ages*. X-Ray evidence may not appear until callus begins to form. Young children are at particular risk.

📁 **Evidence**

Prevalence of fractures in child abuse[7]

A study showed that:

- 58% of the victims of non-accidental fractures were under age three
- 94% of all the non-accidental fractures seen were in children under age three.

Burns

Small round and punched out, are particularly relevant as they can be caused by *cigarettes*.

Scalds

Accidental scalds are splash-shaped. Deliberate ones often show a *glove or stocking* distribution.

Failure to thrive

Failure to thrive may indicate any type of abuse. Particularly suspicious is the child who puts on weight as soon as admitted to hospital.

What to do if abuse is suspected

History

The child may be presented by a parent, health visitor or social worker with either suspected or overt abuse. The child needs to be seen promptly: some are in urgent danger, and in other cases an appointment delay may lead to the child being taken away without being seen. A detailed history of the presenting problem is needed together with the explanations provided by all those involved, including the child's carers and any professionals who are concerned. It is not the GP's role to confront the abuser, but to secure the safety of the child and gather evidence.

Examination

The child should be undressed so that every part of the body can be examined. Embarrassment may be spared older children by replacing some clothing before moving on to the next area. Examination should specifically include the scalp, ears, mouth and genitalia.

Note keeping

Case notes may later be used as evidence, so particular care is needed in their compilation. Details of the history should include details of who said what by way of explanation of the injuries. The clinical findings should be recorded as accurately as possible including the site and size of any bruises and cuts. Diagrams can be very useful.

1. *If abuse is probable*, then the child needs to be in a *safe place*. In practical terms this usually means admission to a paediatric ward. The vast majority of parents will agree with this. If they don't, then there are provisions within the Children Act.
2. *If abuse is possible*, records should be kept just as carefully. It is then recommended that the case be *discussed* with others more experienced such as a paediatrician, the local child protection team, or a National Society for the Prevention of Cruelty to Children (NSPCC) worker.[3] The *NSPCC* have a 24-hour 'hotline' for professionals or members of the public with concerns. Telephone: 0800-800-500.

If not already involved, it is important to also include the *health visitor* in these discussions. Health visitors will often know the families where suspected abuse has occurred, and so will have invaluable insight into the circumstances.

If suspicions of abuse remain it will necessary to inform a *social worker* or the *child protection team* of your concerns. Many departments of social services have specified child protection teams who take responsibility for all child abuse cases in their area. If a child protection team is not available, then their function is performed by social workers.

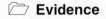 **Evidence**

> **Social services referrals[1]**
>
> In 1991/2 there were:
>
> - 160000 referrals to social services departments
> - 120000 family visits
> - 40000 initial cases conferences
> - 24500 names placed on protection registers.

Confidentiality

The Children Act makes clear what has been considered good practice for some time, namely that the *rights of the child to protection outweigh all other considerations*. The General Medical Council in its booklet *Confidentiality: protecting and providing information* states its position unequivocally.[8] In some situations disclosure of information is proper and necessary, and a GP who decides not to disclose should be prepared to defend the decision.

If you believe a patient to be a victim of neglect or physical, sexual or emotional abuse and that patient cannot give or withhold consent to disclosure, you should give information promptly to an appropriate responsible person or statutory agency, where you believe that the disclosure is in the patient's best interests . . . Such circumstances may arise in relation to children, where concerns about possible abuse need to be shared with other agencies such as social services . . . If, for any reason, you believe that disclosure of information is not in the best interests of an abused or neglected patient, you must still be prepared to justify your decision.

Child protection procedure

Each local authority area has an *area child protection committee* which will set child abuse policy for the area. Policies will vary from place to place, but will be consistent with the Children Act 1989.

In a case of abuse, after due assessment a *child protection conference* will be convened. This will be attended by anyone who might be interested including the social worker, health visitor, teacher, police, parents, etc. The GP is urged to attend and contribute, and can claim a fee for doing so. From this meeting a *key worker* (always a social worker) will be identified, a care plan will be formulated and a decision made whether to place the child's name on the *child protection register*. After this *child protection reviews* will be called to assess progress. At these reviews decisions will be taken concerning

- The need for criminal proceedings
- The need for extra care/supervision
- Whether the child's name should remain on the register
- Whether the case can be closed and the name removed.

The NSPCC is the only voluntary body in this country which has statutory powers under Act of Parliament. Through its 120 or so specialised facilities it can be approached for advice and to perform social work functions.

📄 **Guidelines**   **Role of health services in child protection[3]**

All those working in the field of health have a commitment to protect children, and their participation in inter-agency support to social services departments is essential if the interests of the children are to be safeguarded. Health professionals are major contributors to the inter-agency care of children which extends beyond initial referral and assessment, into child protection conference attendance, participation in planning and the ongoing support of the child and family. There will always be a need for close co-operation with other agencies, including any other health professional involved.

Munchausen's syndrome by proxy (MSP)

The original Munchausen's syndrome was the term applied to people who *fabricate illnesses* and end up having unnecessary investigations and operations. In the proxy form, an adult (usually the mother) either claims symptoms for children, deliberately falsifies tests (e.g. by putting spots of blood in urine specimens) or harms the child usually by poisoning or asphyxiation. The prevalence of MSP is unknown, but is probably relatively low by comparison with all abuse. The first description by Meadow in 1977 reported two cases. By 1993, the same author had knowledge of 300 cases in the UK.[9] The syndrome arises in the under-fives, and usually starts when the child is between one and three months old. Older children may actually come to collude in the deception.

📁 **Evidence**

> **In MSP:[10,11]**
>
> - Death of child – 9%
> - Co-existing abuse of other sorts – 73%
> - Siblings of MSP sufferers:
>
>   11% of the siblings had died in early life
>   17% had been abused in other ways
>   39% had suffered fictitious illnesses.

It is almost invariably the *mothers* who perpetrate this form of abuse. No one psychological diagnosis is responsible. Mothers are often failed nurses or other health professionals, married and of higher social status or more intelligent than their husband. They commonly become very *friendly* with the hospital staff where the child is admitted. The abuse may be due to attention seeking, or may be an attempt to outwit the medical profession.[12] In the typical case

- The child's symptoms defy diagnosis despite being very dramatic
- Symptoms occur only when there is nobody other than mother to witness them
- Tests are invariably normal
- The child's mother is uncommonly chummy with hospital staff, but won't leave the baby for an instant.

Management of MSP is a task for the specialist. The child will need to be separated from the parents as soon as suspicion is aroused.[12] The perpetrator of the abuse will then have to be confronted. This is not an area where the inexperienced should dabble. Whether the diagnosis is confirmed or not, the GP must try to maintain a therapeutic relationship with all family members. Being involved in a highly-charged confrontation situation will jeopardise the GP's future ability to work with the family. The needs of a family following the confirmation of a diagnosis of MSP are considerable.

Child sexual abuse (CSA)

Definitions

Actual or likely sexual exploitation of a child or adolescent. The child may be dependent and/or developmentally immature

OR:

The involvement of dependant developmentally immature children and adolescents in sexual activities that they do not fully comprehend, to which they are unable to give informed consent, and which violate social taboos or family roles.[13]

Prevalence

About 9000 children are on child protection registers in England because of CSA. This is almost certainly an underestimate of the true prevalence.

- A community survey by MORI in 1988 found that 12% of women and 8% of men admitted to being sexually abused in childhood[14]
- Another survey found that 3% of women had experienced actual or attempted penetrative sex in childhood[15]
- At an RCGP meeting reported in 1987, 17% of the women GPs and 9% of the males admitted to being victims of CSA.[16]

Victims

The following factors are statistically associated with CSA. The relationship is not necessarily causal.[17]

- Ever lived without biological father
- Mother employed outside home
- Poor relationship with parent
- Parents in conflict
- Stepfather families
- Chronic physical or psychiatric illness in a parent
- Parent sexually abused in childhood
- Alcohol abuse by parent
- Violence within the family.

The abusers

- Most abusers are *men*, but in 5 to 15% of cases the offence is committed by women acting alone
- A third of offenders cautioned or found guilty of CSA are under 21 years old, and 20% are under 16: half of all CSA offenders start their offending in adolescence[18]
- The majority of CSA occurs within the home: around half of abusers are male family members, and another 12% are male cohabitees or babysitters.[19]

The consequences of CSA

Psychological and physical problems are much commoner in adults who have been sexually abused as children.

- *Physical problems* include pelvic pain, dyspareunia, menstrual disturbance, difficulties in childbirth, non-attendance for cervical screening, sexually transmitted diseases and frequent attendance with minor ailments. In one series 64% of women undergoing laparoscopy for pelvic pain had been sexually abused.[20]

☐ **Evidence**

Physical illness after CSA[21]	
A small study of women who had been sexually abused as children showed:	
Average contacts with non-psychiatric consultants	18
Different non-psychiatrists involved	9
Average surgical operations	8
Normal findings at surgery	70%

- Reluctance to be examined vaginally or have a *cervical smear* is closely associated with CSA in childhood. This is a potentially serious problem as 90% of women diagnosed as having cervical cancer have never had a smear[22]
- *Psychological problems.* Thirty three per cent of adult victims of CSA have psychological problems, compared with 14% of controls.[15] This rises to over 50% for those subjected to penetrative sex. The commonest diagnosis is depression, but low self-esteem, anxiety, obsessional neurosis, sexual problems, marital problems, parenting difficulties and eating disorders are also found.

Detecting CSA

In 39% of cases children themselves report the CSA. This is the most important indicator as most allegations are true.[22] Some are malicious but it is commoner for children to withdraw allegations because they are put under pressure to do so, or because they fear the break-down of their family. In 11% a carer or relative has suspicions. In only 18% of cases the GP is the one who suspects the diagnosis: GPs do not usually have a large role to play in the detection of CSA. The following features may suggest a diagnosis of CSA.[23]

- Aggressive behaviour, tantrums
- Air of detachment 'don't care'
- Excessively compliant, watchful
- Sexually explicit behaviour
- Continual open masturbation, aggressive and inappropriate sex play
- Happy only at school, kept away from school by parent
- Does not join in school activities, few school friends
- Does not trust adults, particularly those who are close
- Unexplained abdominal pains
- Eating problems
- Disturbed sleep, nightmares
- Running away from home, suicide attempts, self-inflicted wounds
- Reverting to younger behaviour, depression, withdrawal
- Secretive and excluding relations with adults.

What to do in suspected CSA

CSA is rarely an emergency in the sense that the child is at grave immediate risk of death.[24] In doubtful cases it is appropriate to discuss with a colleague, paediatrician, child protection team or social worker or the NSPCC. The NSPCC helpline may be particularly useful.

A GP should be non-judgemental in dealing with possible abusers. Abusers have a right to proper care just as does the child. Expressions of disgust are unprofessional and unhelpful.

When confronted with a possible case of CSA it is important to *record what is said and by whom*. Any examination should be cursory only, looking as much for evidence of physical abuse as for signs of CSA. Most CSA victims do not have any physical signs, genital bruising and a torn hymen being features only of extreme abuse involving penetration.

If there is a suspicion of very recent abuse, then the child should be examined by somebody with *forensic experience*, which is more likely to be a police surgeon or a paediatrician. There is no justification in examining the child more than once.

When CSA has been confirmed, the same procedure as for physical abuse is activated.

Other types of abuse

Other categories of child abuse have received less attention than CSA and physical abuse, but they still form a substantial minority of the reasons for inclusion in child protection registers.

Neglect

Neglect is defined as:

> *The persistent or severe neglect of a child, or the failure to protect a child from exposure to any kind of danger, including cold or starvation, or extreme failure to carry out important aspects of care, resulting in the significant impairment of the child's health or development, including non-organic failure to thrive.*[3]

Emotional abuse

Emotional abuse is defined as:

> *Actual or likely severe adverse effect on the emotional and behavioural development of a child caused by persistent or severe emotional ill-treatment or rejection. All abuse involves some emotional ill-treatment. This category should be used where it is the main or sole form of abuse.*[3]

The Children Act 1989

Among its many other provisions, this legislation formalised the basis for the care of abuse victims and their families. It lays great emphasis on the importance of interdisciplinary cooperation and information sharing. There is also provision for using the Act to ensure the safety of an abuse victim.

- *Section 44* gives a social worker power to obtain an emergency protection order to remove a child to a place of safety. This lasts for eight days with a possible extension for a further seven days
- *Section 46* gives a police officer the power to remove a child to a safe place for 72 hours
- *Section 48* gives a police officer power of entry, by force if necessary.

Summary

- Around one million children suffer abuse each year. Most abuse goes undetected and only a fraction of this number appear on child protection registers
- There is a long tradition in the UK of using physical violence against children
- Physical abuse may be life threatening. The child should be removed to a safe place
- Most abusers live in the same household as the abused
- Sexual abuse is rarely life threatening. Urgent specialist attention may however be needed for forensic purposes
- If abuse is suspected it is important to share concerns with other professionals, who may include health visitors, social workers, paediatric specialists or NSPCC workers
- A GP has a professional duty to share information about possible abuse with others
- Child protection is a responsibility of social services departments of local authorities; many have a child protection team to do this work. A GP may be called to contribute to a child protection conference or a child protection review
- Abusers also deserve adequate health care.

Topics for discussion

- A good spanking is the only thing that some children understand
- The law should not interfere with what goes on in the sanctity of the family home
- Communities should be informed of the names and addresses of convicted paedophiles
- Each practice should have a team member with overall responsibility for child protection issues.

References

1. Hobbs C and Wynne J. Child abuse. *General Practitioner*, March 22 1998: 60–2.
2. Meadow R. ABC of child abuse: Epidemiology. *Br Med J* 1989; 298: 727–30.
3. Working Together Under the Children Act 1989. London: HMSO, 1991.
4. Minerva, *Br Med J* 2000; 321: 774.
5. Price J. Non-accidental injury in children: principles of GP management. *Update* 1992; 45: 923–42.
6. Wilson P. Accidental bruising in babies is common on the head and shin. *Medical Monitor* 12 May 1999: 9(13): 28.
7. Hobbs C J. Fractures. *Br Med J* 1989; 298: 1015–18.
8. Confidentiality: Protecting and Providing Information. London: General Medical Council, 2000.
9. Meadow R. False allegations of abuse and Munchausen's syndrome by proxy. *Arch Dis Child* 1993; 68: 444–7.
10. Enoch M D and Trethowan W. Uncommon Psychiatric Syndromes, 3rd edn. London: Butterworths, 1991.
11. Samuels M P, McClaughlin W, Jacobson R R et al. Fourteen cases of imposed upper airways obstruction. *Arch Dis Child* 1992; 67: 162–70.
12. Daniels A. How to recognise Munchausen's by proxy. *Monitor Weekly*, 1993; 3(23): 46–8.

13. Schechter M D and Roberge L. Sexual exploitation. In: Child abuse and neglect: the family and the community. Eds, Helfer R E and Kempe C H. Bellinger: Cambridge, Mass, 1976.
14. Markowe H L J. The frequency of sexual abuse in the UK. *Health Trends* 1988; 20: 2.
15. Hooper P D. Psychological sequelae of sexual abuse in childhood. *Br J Gen Pract* 1990; 40: 29–31.
16. Wilson M S. Sexual abuse of children. *J Roy Coll Gen Pract* 1987; 37: 416.
17. Wilson P and Furnivall J. Sexual abuse in childhood – a problem for life. *Medical Monitor* 1990; 3(38): 35–8.
18. Moore T. Sexual abuse is tip of iceberg. *General Practitioner*, June 17 1994: 53.
19. Diagnosis of Child Sexual Abuse. Standing Medical Advisory Committee. London: HMSO, 1988.
20. Harrop-Griffiths J, Katon W, Walker E et al. The association between chronic pelvic pain, psychiatric diagnosis and childhood sexual abuse. *Obstet Gynecol* 1988; 71: 589–93.
21. Arnold R P, Rogers D and Cook D A G. Medical problems of adults who were sexually abused as children. *Br Med J* 1990; 300: 705–8.
22. Wilson P and Furnivall J. Sexual abuse in childhood – a problem for life. Part 2. *Medical Monitor* 1990; 3(39): 30–2.
23. Cloke C. When to suspect child abuse. *RCGP Connections* (Suppl) 1992; 42: VII.
24. Roberts R. Child sexual abuse and the GP. *The Physician,* October 1988: 691–3.

Child health promotion

Tutorial aims	**The registrar understands the value of child health promotion in primary care, and is able to take an appropriate role in a child health promotion programme.**
Learning objectives	By the end of the tutorial the registrar can: • List the aims of child health promotion • List five items from the six- to eight-week medical • Discuss with parents the significance of a heart murmur • Discuss the role of parents in child health promotion • Test for congenital dislocation of hip • Describe the organisation of a primary care well baby clinic and the roles of the professionals involved • Describe the GP's role when serious congenital abnormality is detected.

In the beginning

For many years there has been state provision for some groups of people to be examined for disease. An example was the Contagious Diseases Act which allowed compulsory examination in garrison towns, and which was not repealed until 1886. In 1906, the school health service was started under local authority control, followed in the 1920s by the child welfare clinics, also under local authority control.[1] During this period infant mortality fell from about 150 per 1000 in 1897 to 70 per 1000 in 1922.[2] The emphasis was on 'provision of medical and especially hygiene advice'.

From this a series of regular medical checks of presumed normal children emerged, leading in 1967 to the publication of the *Sheldon Report*. This report suggested that the work of the child health services should include:[2]

• The performance of routine medicals
• Giving nutrition and hygiene advice
• The detection of defects
• The provision of parental counselling and health education
• Performing immunisations and vaccinations
• The sale of welfare and proprietary foods.

The recommendations of the Sheldon Report were pursued without much question despite there being little evidence that any good was being done. The observed progressive fall in infant mortality can be attributed almost entirely to improvements in living conditions and nutrition rather than to the efforts of doctors or screeners.[1]

In 1989 a joint working party of the British Paediatric Association, the Royal College of General Practitioners, the General Medical Services Committee of the BMA, the Health Visitors Association and the Royal College of Nursing produced a report called *Health for All Children*, or the *Hall Report*.[2] This examined the available evidence and informs the child health programme now in force throughout the UK. The report's third edition in 1996 recommended that the term *child health surveillance* be replaced by *child health promotion*.[3] The three key themes of the Hall Report are[2]

- The content of screening should be determined by the current state of knowledge about the conditions sought, the effectiveness of the test and the availability of programmes for management
- There is good evidence that parents are far better than professionals at detecting a wide range of handicaps at an early stage
- The surveillance programme should include health education.

The value of paediatric screening tests

The value of routine child surveillance has traditionally been challenged because serious disorders in babies often come to attention for reasons not connected with the surveillance, for example

- At the neonatal examination
- As a result of illness or injury requiring consultation with a paediatrician
- Through parental observation
- Detected in the course of a consultation for another problem.[1]

However, child health surveillance is not just about detecting serious disorders. Minor concerns are also prevalent and require proper evaluation and explanation. It is also important to build up good relations between the parents and the child health promotion team.

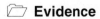 **Evidence**

Physical problems detected by child surveillance[4]

Problems found in

- 58% of children at 14-day check
- 35% of children at 8-week check
- 39% of children at 6–9-month check.

Of the problems detected, 30% needed primary care follow up, and 7% resulted in hospital referral.

📁 **Evidence**

> **Major physical problems detected by child surveillance[5]**
>
> Looking at five conditions – undescended testis, congenital heart disease, squint, hip dysplasia and hearing loss, detected by 18 months
>
> - 21% of children referred, 91% of them from CHS review
> - 12% needed treatment, 84% of them referred after CHS review.

📁 **Evidence**

> **Beneficial paediatric screening tests**
>
> The only medical examinations of which there is strong proof of benefit[2] are:
>
> - Congenital dislocation of hip (CDH)
> - Congenital heart disease
> - Undescended testis (UDT) in boys
> - Laboratory tests
>
>   phenylketonuria (PKU)
>   hypothyroidism.

The monitoring of growth is important, but there must be sufficient expertise in the various techniques of measurement to make it worthwhile. There is evidence that the necessary measuring skills are not universally available.

Hearing and vision are best determined by looking at the child's behaviour with respect to sound and visual stimuli. Looking at the eyes and a hearing distraction test are still recommended, even though there is doubt about the value of the latter.[6]

The child health promotion team

By tradition, doctors through routine medicals have performed most of the surveillance. This is expensive and unproductive, and fails to recognise the abilities of parents and health visitors. It also does not send out good messages to patients about how much doctors trust other primary healthcare workers. Health promotion programmes should be led by health visitors (HVs) with doctors playing only a ceremonial part.

The Hall Report recognises the importance of parents to the surveillance process. Parent-held surveillance records are now virtually universal.

The *aims* of the national child health promotion programme are:[3]

- To ensure that all children have the opportunity to realise their full potential in terms of good health, general well-being and development
- To make sure that remediable disorders are identified and acted upon as early as possible.

Such aims imply that child health promotion is a state of mind, something for a health professional to consider during all contacts with a child. Traditionally many practices have delivered the bulk of child health promotion through a baby clinic, or *Well Baby Clinic*. The use of such clinics is encouraged by the rules governing the child health surveillance fee (see page 80). The value of such clinics includes the facts that:

- All the appropriate staff are in the same place at the same time, and ready for the job in hand
- The regular meeting of the child health promotion team is good for communication
- Ill babies can be excluded
- A doctor is on hand in case of vaccination problems
- The waiting room provides an informal support group for inexperienced parents
- Parents can see that the child health promotion team are all working together.

The timing of checks

A full summary can be found in the Hall Report and subsequent edition.[3] Only those parts indicating GP involvement are given here in detail. Although most of the checks are done by the health visitors, GPs performing paediatric surveillance may be called upon if problems arise.

The timing of the checks continues to be the subject of research. There is now evidence, for instance, that the value of a second neonatal examination is very limited.[7] A single check 24 hours before hospital discharge would detect the vast majority of any significant abnormalities present, but the effect on parental confidence of doing one check rather than two has not been assessed. A second check at 10 days would be better for picking up delayed jaundice and cardiac problems.[8]

At birth, or within the first six hours

This is usually the province of the hospital paediatrician, except for home deliveries and those in a hospital GP unit. A full general physical check is recommended following the same pattern as the six to eight week check. Tests for PKU and hypothyroidism can also be done at this time. Health education advice may include: nutrition; baby care; crying and sleep problems; and safe car transport.

First two weeks

Most GPs will do at least one postnatal visit. GPs working under the general medical services (GMS) contract can claim a fee for postnatal visiting. A doctor or an appropriately trained nurse should check the hips again, but only if there has been no second examination before hospital discharge. This is because there are fears that testing for CDH too frequently can cause damage, particularly in the rare cases of osteogenesis imperfecta. Health education topics may include

- Passive smoking
- Accidents – bathing, scalding, fires
- Immunisation
- Reasons for doing tests for PKU and hypothyroidism (and haemo-globinopathies when indicated).

At six to eight weeks

This is the check needing most GP involvement. It can usefully be combined with the postnatal examination of the mother or coordinated with the first vaccination.

- Check history, review growth, and ask about *parental concerns*
- Enquire specifically about concerns over *hearing, vision and squint*. This can be reinforced by the use of parental checklists
- *Examine* for weight, head circumference, heart murmurs, undescended testes (UDT), CDH and red reflex
- Confirm *vaccination wishes*, and deal with any problems evident at this stage
- Keep the *records* up to date. This will vary with the type of record in use, but generally means making appropriate entries in the parent-held record.

The Children Act 1989 requires professionals to act always in the best interests of the child. This may involve identifying some children as having *special needs* under the terms of the Act. Any such children should be notified to the local authority as possibly eligible for additional social services such as care orders or fostering.

Health education topics may include

- Immunisation
- Dangers of falls, fires, overheating, scalding
- Recognition of illness in babies and what to do.

These issues may be covered in the parent-held record.

At six to nine months

This is primarily the responsibility of the health visitor provided that the essential items of the physical examination can be performed. If this is not the case then a joint GP/HV approach is required. Parental observations and concerns are elicited. Check hearing, UDT, CDH. Health education issues include

- Accident prevention, scalds and burns, falls, problems of increased mobility (though the effectiveness of such advice is doubtful[9])
- Nutrition
- Dental care
- Safety in cars
- Dangers of passive smoking and sunburn.

At eighteen to twenty four months

This check does not require any specific medical input and is appropriately the province of the health visitor. If there are problems contacting the family, however, the GP should try to do the check opportunistically. An assessment of gait and length or height is needed. Health education topics should include:

- Accidents (falls from heights, drowning, poisoning, road safety)
- Nutrition
- Developmental needs

- Language
- Play
- Socialising
- Child behaviour.

Between eight months and fifty four months

The GP should check for *heart abnormalities*. This is usually just a matter of listening to the heart, unless a problem is suspected because of symptoms or unexpected clinical findings. In addition there should be a further check of *testicular descent* if this has not been done since eight months.

It is appropriate to bear in mind the Education Acts of 1981 and 1988 which require that any child who may have *special educational needs* (around 20% of children) should be notified to the local authority at the earliest opportunity. This is a responsibility for anyone who might become aware of a possible need, not just the GP.

At fifty four to sixty six months – school entry

This check is done by the school health service staff. Height, and more detailed vision (Snellen) and hearing ('sweep') tests are done. Other checks or contacts may be required by local policy, for instance in Sheffield there is extra health visitor contact to do with the cot death and postnatal depression prevention programmes.

The Child Health Surveillance (CHS) fee

Since April 1990, GPs who are working under the GMS contract have been able to claim a CHS fee for each child under five years on their list if they obey the rules, namely[10]

- The child must be registered with the doctor for CHS services
- The programme performed must be in accordance with local CHS policy, even though there is evidence that a perfectly adequate system can be run opportunistically by GPs in surgery[11]
- The doctor claiming the fee must be on the health authority's *CHS list*. Methods of getting onto this list vary from place to place. In general, the GP should be able to show evidence of ability to do the checks, and must have the facilities appropriate for doing them. Being on one health authority's list does not automatically qualify you for admission to another's. The CHS fee is about a quarter of the fee for a completed course of infant vaccinations (i.e. £13.45 per child in 2001/02[12]).

The GP contract is quite vague. A GP is required to do (or to delegate) such examinations as are deemed fit by the relevant health authority, and to keep adequate records of what has been done and found.[10] The power is thus all in the hands of the health authority and their henchmen. As an example, the requirements to be on the Sheffield CHS list are

- Proof of experience in child health surveillance or recent hospital training
- Attendance at a course on local CHS policy, lasting two hours
- CHS clinics to be held on a specified half day each week, at a time when

ill people are not in the surgery. Health visitors to be in attendance. There should be sufficient regard to issues of safety, etc.

- The local version of the parent-held CHS record should be used.

The CHS clinical policy which it is necessary to follow is detailed in a health authority document, and this sets out what should be done, when, and by whom.

Diagnosing congenital dislocation of the hip (CDH)

CDH is defined as 'A congenital deformation of the hip joint in which the head of the femur is (or may be) partially or completely displaced from the acetabulum'.[3] It thus includes instability, subluxation and dysplasia, so the term dislocation is misleading.

📂 Evidence

> **Prevalence of CDH[13]**
>
> - Hip instability at birth: 15–20 per 1000
> - Hip instability at one week: 6–8 per 1000.
>
> Ten per cent of unstable hips will persist to show classic signs of dislocation in later infant life, and another 10% will later show evidence of dysplasia and/or subluxation.

The tests used to detect CDH are not particularly good, and the people who do them are often not very proficient.[7] Of the one per 1000 babies who end up needing surgery, 70% are missed by routine screening.[14] Children have to be tested several times, and you can only be sure that a hip is normal when the child is walking with a normal gait.

At-risk groups

Most cases of CDH occur in girls and in firstborn babies. In 60% of cases of CDH, one or more of the following risk factors can be found[13]

- Family history of CDH
- Breech delivery
- Caesarean section delivery
- Other congenital postural deformity, e.g. foot problems
- Oligohydramnios or foetal growth retardation.

📄 Guidelines

When to test for CDH[13]

- Within 24 hours of birth
- Before hospital discharge
- Within the first two weeks of life – may be omitted if two tests already done
- At six to eight weeks
- Between six and nine months
- Between 15 and 21 months
- Gait to be tested at 30 months.

How to test

Trained and committed workers can detect 80–90% of cases of CDH. After the age of six weeks, as the legs extend, the classical signs of CDH become more common. Bilateral CDH is harder to spot than unilateral CDH because there is no normal hip for comparison.

Classical signs

- Leg posture: partial lateral rotation, flexion and abduction
- Limb shortening: above-knee shortening on affected side
- Asymmetry of thighs: skin creases observed from the front
- Flattening of the buttock
- Limitation of abduction: a normal hip in flexion should abduct more than 75°
- Hip instability: specific testing may reveal movement of the femoral head in and out of the acetabulum. *Clicking* or similar in the absence of movement is ligamentous and of no significance.

Gait. Most CDH cases walk at the normal time. However at 18 months 20% are not walking compared to the normal 5%. Any child *not walking at 18 months* should be tested for CDH.

Trendelenburg's sign. At any age over two years, ask the child to stand on one leg. When standing on a leg with CDH, the hip abductors have no fulcrum to hold the pelvis level. This is compensated for by the child leaning over to the affected side, the so-called *Trendelenburg positive*.

Ortolani test

The child is laid on his back with the hip flexed to a right angle and the knees flexed. Starting with the knees together the hips are slowly abducted, and if one is dislocated, somewhere in the 90° arc of abduction the femur slips (forward) back into the acetabulum with a visible and palpable jerk[15]

Barlow test, part 1

The child is laid on his back. The hips are flexed in a right angle and the knees are fully flexed. The middle finger of each hand is closed over the greater trochanter and the thumb of each hand is applied to the inner side of the thigh close to but not quite in the groin. The hips are carried into abduction. With the hips at about 70° of abduction the middle finger of each hand in turn exerts pressure away from the examining couch as if to push the trochanter towards the symphysis pubis. In a normal child no movement occurs. If the hip is dislocated, the greater trochanter and the head of the femur with it can be felt to move in the direction in which the pressure has been applied[5]

Barlow test, part 2

With the hip in the same position as described, the thumb, which is applied over the upper not inner part of the thigh, exerts pressure towards the couch. In a normal child no movement occurs. In a child with CDH the head of the femur can be felt to slip out and come back immediately the pressure is released[15]

After the first month the most important test is limited abduction of the hip when fully flexed.

If on testing it is *suspected* that the child has CDH (which includes a subluxable hip), then there should be a *referral* to a hospital colleague. Tests from a more experienced hand and access to ultrasound imaging will throw more light on the case.

Detecting congenital heart disease

Congenital heart disease is present in about six per 1000 births, but each GP will only see one every five years.[12] Most present *soon after birth*, and two thirds of serious congenital heart disease is detected before the first birthday.[16] Atrial septal defect (ASD) and pulmonary stenosis (PS) may not present until childhood. Minor degrees of ventricular septal defect, ASD or PS while not serious still require *anti-endocarditis prophylaxis*.

A heart murmur is not a disease, it is something that is heard through a stethoscope. Under age 14 a murmur can be heard in all children if the room is quiet enough and especially if the child has recently exercised.[16] *Innocent murmurs* are invariably soft (grade 2/6: easily heard, but faint), but may reach 3/6 (loud, no thrill) in the febrile. Murmurs associated with serious heart disease are:[16]

- Pansystolic or diastolic
- Heard best at the left upper sternal edge, harsh
- Grade 3/6 or greater.

They are also associated with other signs and symptoms:

- Abnormal heart sounds
- Palpable thrill
- Cyanosis
- Breathlessness
- Nasal crepitations, enlarged liver
- Abnormal peripheral pulses
- Poor weight gain.

Non-cardiac chest pain or intermittent cyanosis after bathing or swimming are common in infants and do not indicate heart disease.[14]

Detecting undescended testis (UDT)

📄 Guidelines

When is a testis undescended?[17]

A testis is deemed undescended if the centre of one testis is less than 4 cm below the pubic tubercle, or 2.5 cm in babies under 2.5 kg.

Six per cent of boys are born with one or both testes not in the scrotum. By three months only 1.6% remain undescended; few testes descend after six months. Very rarely, previously descended testes may ascend. Delayed descent may lead to *subfertility*, and there is a 5% chance of *malignant* change in the undescended testis.[18] Orchidopexy before the age of 10 years abolishes the risk of malignant change. If UDT is detected at the eight-week check, it can either be rechecked at three months or else referred straight on to the surgeons. If surgery is needed it should be done around the first birthday. The presence of a hernia makes surgery more likely. Cold hands and too much vigour make testes retract.

Assessing development

It is now recommended that most of the routine developmental checks are done by the health-visiting staff.[3] If a problem is suspected, then the GP will become involved for a second opinion. Health visitors are *highly trained* workers and their opinions should be taken seriously. If they think there is a problem, they are usually correct. A specialist referral will usually be required. A *team approach* to child health promotion requires that the autonomy and skills of each worker are respected. Having proper regard to the opinions of health visitors is important to this end, and the authority and competence of the health visitor will be reinforced as far as the child's parents are concerned.

The only developmental check which the GP is routinely involved with is the one at six to eight weeks, at the time of the GP medical. Some surveillance programmes require more GP checks, but this is because of local policy rather than consistency with the Hall report.

- At eight weeks most babies will be smiling, making noises other than crying, and fixing on and following mother's face
- With the trunk supported, there should be good head control
- In ventral suspension, the arms and legs should be flexed and the head should be held horizontal at least for short periods.

Assessing vision

At eight weeks it is not worth checking vision, but a *red reflex* should be looked for, as should evidence of *squint*. Divergent squint is always abnormal. Convergent squint may be observed for a few months if everything else is all right. The need for early treatment to prevent amblyopia has never been proved.[6] *Parental observation* is the most reliable way of detecting abnormality.[19] Checklists are available to help the parents' assessment

- Does your baby look at you, follow your face and smile back?
- Do the baby's eyes move together?
- Do you think a squint is developing?
- Does your baby turn towards light?

Detecting hearing problems

Parental observation is also the best way of detecting hearing problems.[12] The mean age for the detection of severe deafness by the distraction test is 18 months.[6] Specific questions can be used[19]

- Is your baby startled by sudden loud noises (such as a hand clap or slammed door)? A normal reaction is for the baby's eyes to blink and open
- Are prolonged sounds being noticed? The baby should pause and listen when, for instance, a vacuum cleaner is turned on.

The *at-risk* status of the baby may lead to referral for more detailed testing even if there is no obvious problem. The at-risk group includes[19]

- Family history of childhood deafness
- Congenital abnormalities present, especially craniofacial
- Chromosome abnormalities, especially Down's syndrome
- Neonatal asphyxia
- Ventricular haemorrhage
- Maternal infections: cytomegalovirus; rubella; toxoplasma
- Birth weight under 1.5 kg.

Summary

- The routine medical examination of supposedly normal babies has a long tradition, but there is limited evidence for its effectiveness
- Current child health promotion recommendations are in general consistent with the available evidence, and reinforced by the payment of the CHS fee to GPs
- Child health promotion is a team game, in which the child's parents are key players
- Health promotion should be on the agenda for all contacts with children
- The well baby clinic is an ideal format for delivering child health promotion
- Health visitors are an invaluable resource and should properly be responsible for most of the routine child checks
- Detecting CDH requires skill and dedication, and most cases are missed at first
- A heart murmur almost never indicates serious heart disease in a child
- For detecting problems with vision and hearing, parental observation is particularly useful.

🗨 Topics for discussion

- Child health promotion is a normal part of general medical services and so the CHS fee should be scrapped
- Most mothers know when their baby is abnormal, but most grandparents do not
- Euthanasia should be available for severely abnormal babies
- How can parents be integrated into the child health promotion team?
- In the light of current demographic trends, what changes in child health promotion might be necessary in the next 20 years?

📖 References

1. Hannay D. Future of General Practice and Child Health. Sheffield: University of Sheffield, 1989.
2. Polnay L and Hall D M B. Child Health Surveillance. *BMJ* 1989; 299: 1351–3.
3. Hall D B M, ed. Health for all children, 3rd edn (HFAC3). Joint working party of British Paediatric Association, General Medical Services Committee, Royal College of General Practitioners, Royal College of Nursing, Health Visitors' Association. Oxford: Oxford University Press, 1996.
4. Hampshire A J, Blair M E, Crown N S *et al.* Are child health surveillance reviews just routine examinations of normal children? *Br J Gen Pract* 1999; 49: 981–5.
5. Hampshire A J, Blair M E, Crown N S *et al.* Is pre-school child health surveillance an effective means of detecting key physical abnormalities? *Br J Gen Pract* 1999; 49: 630–3.
6. Robinson R. Effective screening in child health. *BMJ* 1998; 316: 1–2.
7. Hall D B M. The role of the routine neonatal examination. *BMJ* 1999; 318: 619–20.
8. Wilson P. When should babies be examined?. *Medical Monitor* 1993; 6(5): 25.
9. Kendrick D, Marsh P, Fielding K and Miller P. Preventing injuries in children: cluster randomised controlled trial in primary care. *BMJ* 1999; 318: 980–3.
10. National Health Service (General Medical Services) Regulations London: HMSO, 1992.
11. Houston H L A, Santos K and Davis R H. Opportunistic developmental surveillance in general practice. *Br J Gen Pract* 1990; 40: 230–2.
12. Medeconomics database. June 2001.
13. Screening for the Detection of Congenital Dislocation of the Hip. London: Standing Medical Advisory Committee, 1986.
14. McKee L. Screening babies for hip dislocation is not effective. *BMJ* 1998; 316: 1265.
15. Sharrard W. in *The Newborn*. Pulse Reference, March 17 1984.
16. Abrams S and Walsh K. Murmurs: a cause for concern? *The Practitioner* 1997; 241: 663–6.
17. Reilly H. Is one testes test enough? *General Practitioner*, July 15 1994: 23.
18. The examination of the testes in childhood. Sheffield: FHSA/DHA, 1989.
19. Clinical Policy for Child Health Surveillance and Immunisation (Pre-school). Sheffield Health Authority and Sheffield FHSA. 2nd Edition. February 1993.

Chronic fatigue syndrome (CFS)

Tutorial aim	**The registrar can negotiate a management plan for a patient with CFS.**
Learning objectives	By the end of the tutorial the registrar can: • Recall three diagnostic criteria for CFS • Recall four differential diagnoses for CFS • Display an appropriate attitude towards a patient who has CFS • Help a patient with CFS choose suitable treatment • Discuss the role of CFS self-help groups • Predict the possible future needs of a patient with CFS.

Introduction

Chronic fatigue syndrome is a major cause of illness and disability.[1] The typical victim is an active intelligent young woman who is reduced by CFS to a shadow of her former self. Because CFS can be so disabling, because it affects people in the prime of life, and because there is no reliable cure, the disease and its victims repeatedly hit the headlines. However, many medical authorities dispute that CFS actually exists. To the victim this has overtones of professional negligence if not misogyny. The caring GP will be reluctant to make a diagnosis of CFS until it is clear that the fatigue is not being caused by the myriad other, and possibly curable, alternative illnesses.

Statistics

Tiredness is very common.

• Up to a third of people at any one time say they have had fatigue for the last month or more[2]
• Just over 10% of all people attending their GP complain of fatigue[3] (fatigue is, after respiratory problems, the commonest symptom complained of[4])
• Patients will report only about one in 400 episodes of fatigue to their GP[5]
• A GP with a list size of 2000 can expect 26 presentations a year for fatigue as the main symptom, and 150 more who have fatigue as well as other symptoms.[4]

The differential diagnosis of fatigue is huge. Indeed fatigue is probably a feature of all illness with the possible exception of mania. In about three quarters of cases the cause of the fatigue turns out to be *psychosocial*, and in about a tenth a physical cause is found.[6] Some of the rest will be diagnosed as having CFS.

📁 **Evidence**

Differential diagnosis of tiredness[6]	
• Psychosocial problems (75%)	
• Physical (10%)	
anaemia	hypothyroidism
medication	cardiovascular disease
chronic neurological disorders	chronic kidney or liver disease
malignancy (under 1%)	postviral fatigue
• Unexplained (includes CFS) (15%)	

CFS has a lot of different names including *neuraesthenia, Royal Free disease, yuppie flu* and *myalgic encephalomyelitis (ME)*. Some descriptions of the illness are quite old, dating back to 1781.[7] Diagnostic criteria were formulated only in 1978[7] and the current consensus was agreed only in 1991,[8] which makes old sources unreliable and estimates of prevalence open to dispute. The Royal Free epidemic of 1955 was almost certainly caused by mass hysteria.[7]

Myalgic encephalomyelitis is the most popular name with patients, and indeed ME is the only disease legally recognised in Britain.[7] ME is also the term favoured by most of the relevant self-help organisations, even though there is no evidence that encephalitis plays any part in the symptoms.[9] The medical establishment currently favours the term chronic fatigue syndrome.[8]

Estimates of the prevalence of CFS range from three in 100 000 to one in 1000,[7] a thirty-five-fold difference.

- The ME Association (a self-help and campaigning group) estimate that there are 80 000 to 120 000 cases in the UK and 500 000 cases worldwide[7]
- A community survey of adults in south-east England found that 0.2% of respondents considered themselves to have CFS, but 1% reported some of the diagnostic features[3]
- Other estimates put the prevalence as high as 2.6%.[9]

CFS is found in all social classes and ethnic groups. The only known demographic risk factor is that CSF is commoner in women.[10]

Nobody knows what causes CFS. It may not even be a single condition, but a group of symptoms which can result from a number of different causes or combinations of these. A mass of research data exists, the results of which have suggested different possible causative mechanisms. However, little of the research is beyond criticism, and the authoritative consensus remains that the cause(s) of CFS is unknown.[8] Accordingly there are no blood or other tests which will reliably confirm a diagnosis of CFS. Similarly there are no completely reliable physical signs.

🖹 Guidelines

Suggested causes of CFS[11]

- Viral infection
- Psychological disorder
- Stress and life events
- Personality
- Abnormalities of the hypothalamo-pituitary-adrenal axis
- Abnormalities of central 5-hydroxytryptamine function
- Abnormalities in cerebral blood flow.

There is good evidence that *infection* with the Epstein-Barr virus, viral hepatitis and meningitis can *trigger* CFS.[11] After a bout of glandular fever, up to 10% of patients develop symptoms like CFS.[1] Chronic consequences from other viral triggers are less likely, and tend to be more common in patients who had symptoms of fatigue before they contracted the virus: some people seem *predisposed* to CFS which is then triggered by a viral infection.

Stress and a*dverse life events* certainly make an individual more likely to get CFS after a viral trigger.[11] Three fifths of the victims of CHS have *no previous psychiatric diagnoses*, but the illness itself can cause significant stress and sometimes leads to depression.[1] The minority of patients who get referred to specialist clinics for tiredness are a selected group who are likely to have more severe symptoms: they tend to be perfectionist and over-achieving,[11] but this is probably not true of the generality of less severe CFS seen in primary care. Research carried out on referred populations can be misleading.

Tiredness is common in all social classes, and especially in women who have children aged under six years; this is not surprising as young women with families work an average 77 hours a week.[5]

All the recommended *treatments are disappointing*. Many authorities dispute that CFS is a discrete disease entity at all, and regard it as a variant of depression[12] with which it shares many features.

Diagnosing CFS

As far as a patient with CFS is concerned, making the diagnosis is seen as the most *helpful* thing which a GP can do.[13] This requires having positive diagnostic criteria, and at the same time having sufficient regard to the differential diagnosis to be able to exclude other problems. The criteria given in the box are derived from a consensus reached at a conference in Oxford in 1991. They are not the only criteria in use. The Americans use the criteria from the US Centers for Disease Control and Prevention (1994) which importantly do not require mental fatigue to be present. In the US CFS is seen more as a physical illness, and this affects attitudes, treatments and prevalence statistics.

📄 **Guidelines**   **Oxford diagnostic criteria for CFS[10]**

- Severe, disabling fatigue of at least six months' duration that affects both physical and mental functioning and is present for more than 50% of the time

- Other symptoms, particularly myalgia and sleep and mood disturbance may be present.

- Exclusions:

   Active, unresolved or suspected disease likely to cause fatigue
   Psychotic, melancholic or bipolar depression (but not uncomplicated major depression)
   Psychotic disorders
   Dementia
   Anorexia or bulimia nervosa.

The Oxford diagnostic criteria were developed primarily to aid in research into CFS, and are possibly too narrow for clinical use because of their exclusions.

CFS is primarily characterised by persistent or relapsing physical and mental fatigue, lasting over six months, not relieved by rest and readily distinguishable by sufferers from normal fatigue. Symptoms are often brought on by bouts of physical or mental activity, usually after a delay of a day or so, or the day after drinking alcohol.[1] Other symptoms associated with the fatigue are less specific, and may alter with time. The commonest include[1]

- Muscle pain
- Joint pain with no evidence of inflammation
- Sore throat, tender lymph glands
- Headache
- Dizziness and vertigo
- Feeling feverish
- Paraesthesiae
- Altered perception of sound and light
- Symptoms of irritable bowel syndrome or food intolerance
- Palpitation, feelings of breathlessness
- Tender 'trigger points'
- Poor concentration and short-term memory
- Mood swings, panic attacks, depression
- Sleep is often disturbed and unrefreshing.

This is a considerable list, and the symptoms could just as well be found in numerous other illness presentations which GPs find difficult to manage. The refusal by some doctors to accept the existence of CFS may well be based on exasperation.

The diagnosis of CFS is *based primarily on the history*, and on the clinician being prepared to accept that the diagnosis is possible. A clinical examination is not usually helpful. A few investigations designed to exclude other diagnoses can be of help, with the proviso that a diagnosis by exclusion is rarely satisfying to a patient, and the delay in getting the results back can cause anxiety. And, of course, if enough tests are done, eventually one will show an abnormality.[14]

📄 **Guidelines**   **Blood tests in CFS[1]**

- Full blood count
- Inflammatory markers – erythrocyte sedimentation rate or C-reactive protein
- Urea and electrolytes, creatinine
- Liver function tests
- Thyroid function tests
- Glucose
- Creatine kinase.

The role of the GP

Most GPs will have had the experience of a consultation with a young articulate female patient who has attended having diagnosed herself as having CFS (or more likely ME). Whether you 'believe in' CFS or not, the patient's problems still have to be addressed. It is clear that CFS is a complex interaction of cerebral dysfunction, trigger factors and social attitudes.[9] Of all doctors, GPs should be aware that trying to decide whether symptoms are physical or psychological is futile: all physical symptoms have psychological consequences and vice versa.

Acceptance

Many patients with CFS do not feel that their GP takes them seriously. Doctors quite commonly evade their patients' ideas, and this is twice as common with women as with men patients.[5] This is not surprising in CFS if some GPs dispute its existence. It is nevertheless professionally incumbent on the practitioner to present the patient with a reasonable treatment plan. If the GP feels that the reason for the symptoms is not CFS, then alternative diagnoses should be discussed. Being rude or dismissive is not justified when in reality the problem is that the GP is unable to reach a diagnosis.

Diagnosis

The recent high profile of CFS means that it is probably being over-diagnosed. Disease processes within the differential diagnosis of CFS are many and varied, and include some important ones. The use of proper diagnostic criteria should enable a positive diagnosis to be made. In patients who do not have CFS, equal rigour must be employed in making and negotiating an alternative diagnosis.

Activity

Controlled exercise substantially improves the symptoms of CFS.[15] This recommendation is sometimes resisted, especially among sufferers who consider CFS to be a purely physical disorder. With inactivity muscles rapidly become deconditioned, and once deconditioned even minor exertion will cause fatigue and pain. The best bet seems to be regular brief exercise which falls just short of producing a severe reaction. This can be a bit of a lottery as tolerance to exertion may well alter from day to day. For each patient a baseline of activity must be found which does not provoke a relapse: the baseline can then be increased upon by small tolerable amounts. Half an hour's limb movement and light jogging twice a day has been suggested.[16] More intense exercise programmes are also associated with benefit, but the drop-out rate is higher.[10]

📁 **Evidence**

> **Graded exercise in CFS[17]**
>
> A study of 148 patients attending a CFS clinic and fulfilling the Oxford criteria who achieved a satisfactory outcome
>
> - Normal care – medical assessment, advice, information booklet encouraging graded activity and positive thinking, 6%
> - Intervention – above plus evidence-based explanations of symptoms, tailored graded exercise programme, educational information pack and two face-to-face follow-up sessions totalling three hours, 69%
>
> Increased intervention by telephone calls or extra face-to-face sessions did not further improve the outcome.

Dietary advice

Sufferers from CFS are nearly always *intolerant of alcoholic drinks*;[12] the intolerance may be to the alcohol itself or to other ingredients. For other patients *caffeine, eggs, wheat or cow's milk* may worsen symptoms. Many patients presenting with CFS will have tried exclusion diets before attending: some of these diets will have been so severe as to be nutritionally unsound.

Efamol marine, a combination of marine oils and evening primrose oil is supposed to help 80% of CFS sufferers.[12] It cannot be prescribed for this indication, but is available (at a price) from health food shops. Trials using just *evening primrose oil* have given conflicting results.[10]

Medication

Sleep disturbance and depression can be helped by *tricyclic antidepressants*. The dosages suggested are lower than antidepressant doses, typically 25 to 50 mg a day.[12,18] There may be patient *resistance* to the idea of taking anti-depressants as some will think the doctor is implying that the symptoms are imaginary. Getting the patient onto suitable medication will require tact and diplomacy, qualities for which GPs are justly famous. There is insufficient evidence to recommend antidepressants of any type for the treatment of other CFS symptoms.[10]

Gut overgrowth with c*andida albicans* can be responsible for abdominal bloating, disturbance of bowel action and perianal itching. *Nystatin* or *amphotericin* taken orally may be effective and is worth a try.

Other suggested treatments include corticosteroids and oral nicotinamide adenine dinucleotide (NAHD). None are of proven effectiveness.[10] One small trial has found benefit from the use of magnesium injections, in the absence of proven magnesium deficiency. Injections of IgG may be of limited benefit, but there is a high risk (over 80%) of side effects. Other forms of immunotherapy are of unproven benefit.[10]

Talking treatments

The other treatment (apart from exercise) which has been shown substantially to improve symptoms in CFS is *cognitive behavioural therapy*, with a number needed to treat of only two for return to normal function after a year.[10] This result was achieved using highly skilled therapists working in specialised centres and must be compared with the natural history of fatigue: with ordinary GP care, half of patients complaining of fatigue will feel better six months later.[4]

Evidence

Counselling and cognitive behavioural therapy in CFS[19, 20]

In an uncontrolled trial of patients presenting in general practice with chronic fatigue

- Counselling and cognitive behavioural therapy were equally effective
- After six months average fatigue scores had fallen from 23 to 15, and nearly half of patients no longer fulfilled the entry diagnostic criteria for fatigue
- Costs (£164 for cognitive behavioural therapy and £109 for counselling at 2001 prices) were not found to differ at a level of significance.

Referral

Referral is particularly useful if a diagnosis other than CFS is being considered. Many patients will welcome the opportunity to ensure that no horrid diagnosis is being missed. Some of the more esoteric biochemical and serological associations with CFS are in any case best assessed by a doctor who is more familiar with them than the average GP. Only 2% of patients presenting to GPs with fatigue get referred.[4]

Guidelines

Reasons to refer to a specialist include[11]

- Elderly patient (CFS is rare in the elderly, and a sinister diagnosis commoner)
- History of foreign travel (possible exotic infection)
- Weight loss (CFS is associated with weight gain)
- Neurological signs present
- Difficulty walking
- Pyrexia of unknown origin
- Abnormal investigations
- Patient request.

It is not immediately clear who would be the *appropriate specialist* for the referral of a suspected case of CFS. I have always received an excellent service from the local infectious diseases unit, but I am really not sure if theirs is the appropriate expertise or if they are just an agreeable and helpful bunch of doctors. Perhaps an immunologist or clinical pathologist would be a suitable alternative. The personal qualities of the specialist are at least as important as their specific technical skills. An increasing number of clinics dedicated to CFS are being set up, most of them in the private sector. A referral might be appropriate when the search for an alternative diagnosis has been abandoned. If treatments such as counselling or cognitive behavioural therapy are not available in primary care, specialised services may be offered at a secondary care clinic.

An action plan

Most patients who present to their GP complaining of fatigue will not have CFS. By far the majority will be either depressed or anxious. Patients with psychological fatigue are often resistant to the idea that their physical symptoms are produced by psychological problems. The anxious are worried about serious or even terminal disease and do not want to be fobbed off without further investigation. The depressed will believe it is all their own fault and will want to take personal responsibility for their plight. An action plan could be as follows:

- Ask about other symptoms associated with *depression*: sleep disturbance, guilt, anhedonia, etc.
- Ask also about sources of *stress*: this may not be too helpful as most people have got stresses of some sort, but identifying a particular stress can be a good way of convincing a patient that there is indeed a logical reason for how they feel
- Ask about symptoms which might indicate *organic disease*, such as weight loss, polyuria
- If there is no reason to suspect other pathology, try to elicit a *positive history* of CFS using the diagnostic criteria
- *Blood tests* may be useful. The ones suggested above can be supplemented if some aspect of history suggests a particular pathology
- *Consider referral*. CFS can be a long and troublesome illness. If no alternative diagnosis can be reached or management plan agreed, then all sufferers deserve access to a suitable specialist opinion
- Consider *medication*. The use of tricyclics has already been mentioned. Some patients get a lot of pain and need analgesia. Sometimes a low dose of tricyclic will help with the pain
- Arrange a system of *follow up*. The GP with a patient with CFS has two options: either agree a series of consultations in advance, or the patient will present each new symptom as it arises to any doctor who happens to be available. A balance has to be found between properly exploring new symptoms, and keeping in mind the context of the CFS. Patients with CFS need *continuity of care* from a doctor with whom they can see eye to eye. It is poor GP practice to refuse this responsibility and to allow a patient to drift rudderless around colleagues.

Self-help groups

Myalgic Encephalomyelitis Association
PO Box 8
Stanford-le-Hope
Essex SS17 0AH
Telephone: 01375 642466

Action for ME
PO Box 1302
Wells, BA5 1YE
Telephone: 01749 670799

As can be seen from their titles, both the above prefer the term myalgic encephalomyelitis to chronic fatigue syndrome. Their literature shows a clear preference for the physical theories about the cause of CFS, with much guidance about rest/exercise, dietary supplements and vitamins. They are also very keen that sufferers receive specialist input for their problems. Participation in a self-help group is associated with a *worse prognosis* for the CFS,[13] but this may be no more than a reflection of the type of people who join self-help groups, and perhaps suggests that the more severely affected and those making little progress are more likely to become involved.

The prognosis of CFS

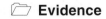 **Evidence**

> **Outlook for 'tiredness'[4]**
>
> A study from general practice of patients presenting with tiredness:
>
> - About half had improved after six months
> - Poorer outlook was associated with
>
>   being a woman
>   symptoms at presentation for more than three months
>   history of emotional illness.

The chance of getting over CFS is related to how bad it is. Work on CFS tends to be derived from the experience of specialised clinics where presumably the more severe cases are referred. These suggest that up to 50% of adults but up to 94% of children with CFS improve over six-year follow up. However, only 6% return to completely normal functioning.

Outcome is influenced by the presence of *psychiatric disorder*, and *beliefs* about causation and treatment.[10] Those who do best are those who:

- Are less severely affected
- Have not had their symptoms for as long
- Are less likely to attribute their symptoms to a physical cause
- Feel a greater sense of control over their symptoms.[21]

There have been no reported mortalities from CFS.

Summary

- Tiredness or fatigue is a feature of nearly all illness
- The prevalence of chronic fatigue syndrome may be as high as one in 40. It is found in all social groups, but is commoner in women
- Many symptoms have been attributed to CFS. Whatever other symptoms are present, all sufferers have excessive levels of mental and physical fatigue which has been present for more than six months

- The existence of CFS is not universally accepted. It shares a lot of clinical features with depression
- There are no tests which will confirm CFS
- The GP's most valued contribution to care is to accept the diagnosis
- Only graded exercise and cognitive behavioural therapy have been shown to improve the outlook in CFS
- The outlook for severe protracted CFS is not good: only a fraction of patients secure a complete recovery
- Sufferers who hold the view that CFS is primarily a physical problem have a worse prognosis.

🗨 Topics for discussion

- What are the advantages and disadvantages of encouraging patients with CFS to seek the advice of alternative practitioners?
- The Teachers' Pension Scheme will no longer accept CFS for the purposes of early retirement on the grounds of ill health. What are the implications of this decision?
- Patients with CFS do better if they accept that it has a strong psychological dimension. Would medical practitioners do better to reinforce this by regarding CFS as a type of depression?
- To what extent should each individual symptom of CFS be investigated?
- The NHS should make sure that a specialised CFS clinic is readily available for all sufferers.

📖 References

1. Pinching A J. Chronic fatigue syndrome. *Prescribers' Journal* 2000; 40(2): 99–106.
2. Ridsdale L. Tired all the time. *BMJ* 1991; 303: 1490–1.
3. Pawlikowska T, Chalder T, Hirsch S R et al. Population based study of fatigue and psychological distress. *BMJ* 1994; 308: 763–6.
4. Ridsdale L, Evans A, Jerrett W et al. Patients with fatigue in general practice: a prospective study. *BMJ* 1993; 307: 103–6.
5. Ridsdale L, Evans A, Jerrett W et al. Patients who consult with tiredness: frequency of consultation, perceived causes of tiredness and its association with psychological distress. *Br J Gen Pract* 1994; 44: 413–16.
6. Gambrill E C and Mead M. 'Tired all the time' *Update* 1994; 49: 233–5.
7. Archer M I. The post-viral syndrome: a review. *J Roy Coll Gen Pract* 1987; 37: 212–14.
8. Straus S E. Chronic fatigue syndrome. *BMJ* 1996; 313: 831–2.
9. Thomas P K. The chronic fatigue syndrome: what do we know? *BMJ* 1993; 306: 1557–8.
10. Reid S, Chalder T, Cleare A et al for "*Clinical Evidence*" Chronic fatigue syndrome. *BMJ* 2000; 320: 292–6.
11. Cleare A J and Wessely S C. Chronic fatigue syndrome: an Update. *Update* 1996; 53: 61–9.
12. M.E. – Information for doctors. Wells: *M.E. Action Campaign*, 1991.
13. Elliott H. Use of formal and informal care among people with prolonged fatigue: a review of the literature. *Br J Gen Pract* 1999; 49: 131–4.
14. Anon. Editor's choice: Are you normal? *BMJ* 1997; 314.
15. Fulcher K Y and White P D. Randomised controlled trial of graded exercise in patients with chronic fatigue syndrome. *BMJ* 1997; 314: 1647–52.

16. Haines P. Doctors unravel M E puzzle. *General Practitioner* September 24 1993: 37.
17. Powell P, Bentall R P, Nye F J and Edwards R H T. Randomised controlled trial of patient education to encourage graded exercise in chronic fatigue syndrome. *BMJ* 2001; 322: 387–90.
18. Cooper N. What does ME mean to me? *Maternal and Child Health* 1992; 17(1): 21–4.
19. Ridsdale L, Godfrey E, Chalder T *et al*. Chronic fatigue in general practice: is counselling as good as cognitive behaviour therapy? A UK randomised trial. *Br J Gen Pract* 2001; 51: 19–24.
20. Chisholm D, Godfrey E, Ridsdale L *et al*. Chronic fatigue in general practice: economic evaluation of counselling versus cognitive behaviour therapy. *Br J Gen Pract* 2001; 51: 15–18.
21. Marshall J. Prognosis is often poor in chronic fatigue syndrome. *Medical Monitor* 26 June 1996: 42.

Coping with cholesterol

Tutorial aim

The registrar understands the role of cholesterol in the prevention of coronary heart disease.

Learning objectives

By the end of the tutorial the registrar can:

- Discuss cholesterol in relation to other risk factors for coronary heart disease
- Describe how to take a blood sample for measuring cholesterol
- Demonstrate the use of the Joint British Recommendations
- Quote target cholesterol levels for coronary heart disease (CHD) prevention
- Discuss with a patient the advantages and disadvantages of cholesterol screening
- Describe the appropriate use of statins in primary care
- Describe the importance of statins to the Primary Care Group/Trust.

The importance of cholesterol

Heart attacks killed 166 753 people in the United Kingdom (UK) in 1992.[1] In addition there are over two million people in the UK who have CHD.

- 150 000 heart attack survivors
- 1 400 000 angina sufferers
- 500 000 people with heart failure, and
- 22 000 coronary artery bypass grafts and 14 000 coronary arterioplasties are performed each year.[2]

Even though the death rate from CHD has been declining for 20 years, it is by far the commonest cause of death.

- CHD is responsible for 27% of all male deaths and 21% of all female deaths[3]
- CHD is the biggest cause of premature death: one in six men and one in 15 women die from CHD before the age of 75[4]
- In 1991/92 in the UK, 53 million working days were lost because of CHD, over 10% of all days lost to sickness. This cost £463 million in sickness benefits, and £3 billion in lost production.[4]

Cholesterol levels have a *linear relationship* with CHD risk both within and between populations.[5] In the absence of other risk factors, the death rate from CHD in men in the lowest quintile of cholesterol is, at 26 per 100 000 per year, only a quarter of the death rate of those in the highest quintile.[6]

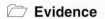 **Guidelines**

Cholesterol levels in the UK population[7]

Under 5.2 mmol/L	5%
5.2 to 6.4 mmol/L	40%
6.5 to 7.8 mmol/L	25%
Over 7.8 mmol/L	10%

People with the highest cholesterol levels run the highest risk of having a heart attack, but there are many more people in the moderate risk group so that more heart attacks occur in this group.

In 1997 the total expenditure on lipid-lowering drugs was £134 million (of which £113 million was spent on statins) up from £20 million in 1993.[3]

The NHS *National Service Framework for Coronary Heart Disease* requires primary care teams to identify and modify the risk factor in people with a heart disease risk of over 3% a year. Primary Care Groups/Trusts are required to adopt strategies to achieve this target.

Who should have their cholesterol tested?

There are many known risk factors for CHD,[8] and by itself cholesterol is not a very good way of predicting a heart attack.[3] The people who should be tested are those in whom reducing cholesterol might do some good. It is currently recommended that people with a CHD risk of 30% or more over 10 years (or 3% per year) deserve preventive intervention, and that as resources allow the work should be extended to all those with a risk of 1.5% per year.[9]

Evidence

> **Population CHD risk[10]**
>
> According to a study from Scotland of people aged 35 to 64
>
> - 2.2% have a CHD risk of over 3% a year
> - 13% have a CHD risk of over 1.5% a year
>
> The potential scope for CHD-lowering interventions is enormous.

Raised CHD risk – primary prevention

The evidence that patients with raised cholesterol but without CHD benefit from treatment has taken a long time coming. Early research showed reduced coronary mortality, but all-cause mortality was unchanged: accident and suicide deaths were higher in treatment groups, an anomaly which has still not been completely explained.

The first indication of the benefit of artificial cholesterol lowering in primary prevention was revealed by meta-analysis, suggesting that the early trials were not big enough to have sufficient statistical power.[11] All this changed with the publication of the *West of Scotland study (WOSCOPS)*,[12] a controlled trial of 6600 men aged 45 to 64 who did not have CHD, but who did have a raised cholesterol, median 7 mmol/L. The study demonstrated that treatment with a statin, pravastatin, over a five-year period produced a reduction in heart attacks of 31% and a reduction in all-cause deaths of 22%, though this latter did not reach statistical significance. Curiously, the effect did not depend on the age or the smoking habits of the subjects.

Further work on the data[13] suggests that the level of benefit is proportionately the same for all base-line levels of risk: *those with increased risk get increased benefit*, but in the very low-risk subjects the benefit conferred by pravastatin is tiny.

Work done on data from the Framingham project has led to joint recommendations from the British Cardiac Society, the British Hyperlipidaemia Association, the British Hypertension Society and the British Diabetic Association.[9] With the backing of such august groups, these recommendations must be taken seriously. They can be regarded as 'truth' for the time being.

These *Joint British Recommendations on prevention of coronary heart disease in clinical practice* include charts to estimate CHD risk (non-fatal MI and coronary death) in primary prevention.[9] Risk can be calculated according to age and sex, exposure to tobacco smoke (total lifetime exposure rather than just current smoking habits), blood pressure, and the presence or absence of diabetes. Risks of 30 and 15% over 10 years are indicated.

📄 Guidelines

Primary prevention of CHD[9]

Intervention is recommended where CHD risk is 30% or greater over 10 years (3% per year). This should be extended to people with a risk of over 15% as resources allow.

The Joint British Recommendation charts recognise that they underestimate CHD risk for

- Family history of premature CHD (men <55 years, women <65 years): multiply risk by 1.5
- Raised triglyceride
- Impaired glucose tolerance (but not diabetes)
- Premature menopause
- Patients approaching the next age category.

The charts do not give figures for patients over 70. This is because there is insufficient research evidence available for older people, and in the elderly cholesterol levels seem less important in determining CHD risk. However the rate of CHD rises with age, and so older people are at highest risk of an event: it is probably only a matter of time before research will plug this knowledge gap. The tables have also been criticised for excluding social class in their calculations. The 'acceptable' risk of myocardial infarction of 3% a year could be seen as a bit high.

An alternative form of the charts is available as the new *Sheffield tables.*[10] These are based on the same Framingham data, and also need a ratio of total cholesterol to HDL for their use. They similarly underestimate risk for some categories of patient:

- Left ventricular hypertrophy (LVH) on ECG (double risk – add 20 years to age)
- Family history of CHD (add six years)
- Familial hyperlipidaemia
- British Asian patients.

There is little point in measuring everyone's cholesterol, and it is not recommended as a screening procedure.[3] Having a cholesterol test seems to have no motivational effect at least as far as smoking and diet are concerned.[14]

Familial raised cholesterol

Around one in 500 of the UK population have familial hypercholesterolaemia, and another one in 200 have other familial hyperlipidaemias. The levels of serum lipid found in these groups is frequently exceedingly high, so that a total cholesterol of over 10 mmol/L would not be unusual. These people are at particular risk of CHD independent of other risk factors, and benefit from lipid-lowering treatment.

📄 **Guidelines**

Identifying familial hypercholesterolaemia[9]

People who are aged over 18 and who have a first-degree relative (siblings or parents) who has premature CHD or other atherosclerotic disease (men under 55, women under 65) may have familial hypercholesterolaemia. They should have their cholesterol measured, and be treated as for secondary prevention with aspirin and a statin.

Secondary Prevention

Pre-existing CHD is a powerful predictor of future CHD events, and the case for reducing cholesterol in these patients is very strong.[3] Patients who have had a myocardial infarct, or who have angina or peripheral vascular disease should have their cholesterol level measured.[4]

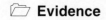 **Evidence**

The Scandinavian simvastatin survival study (4S)[15]

4444 patients with CHD treated with simvastatin followed up for 5.5 years
33% reduction in coronary events
30% reduction in total deaths
Looked at another way, the number needed to treat (NNT) over five years using a statin in patients with CHD is 11 per coronary event, and 27 per coronary death.

Patients with some other diseases should be treated as though they already have CHD. They should be taking aspirin, and their cholesterol should be measured and if necessary reduced with a statin.[9]

- Other major arteriosclerotic disease – stroke, TIA
- Sustained hypertension (systolic ≥160 mmHg *or* diastolic ≥100 mmHg) or with hypertensive end-organ damage
- Diabetes mellitus
- Renal dysfunction.

Measuring cholesterol

What to measure Cholesterol is deposited to form atheromatous plaques. Low density lipoprotein (LDL) is the major transporter of cholesterol in the blood and this subfraction largely accounts for the close relationship of total cholesterol levels to CHD.[5] On the other hand, high density lipoprotein (HDL) is inversely related to CHD risk. Triglyceride levels are elevated in a number of lipid disorders, but though they may cause pancreatitis, their role in CHD is not clear.

If CHD is already present, then total cholesterol should be measured. In the absence of CHD (primary prevention) then total cholesterol and HDL should be measured. The Joint British Recommendations and the Sheffield tables use total cholesterol divided by HDL to assess risk. Both total cholesterol and HDL can be assessed from a non-fasting blood sample.[9]

Taking the Sample A number of things are known to alter a cholesterol assay[8]

- *Posture* may alter the reading by up to 10%. Levels fall significantly on sitting, and fall further on lying down
- *Occluding* the vein for more than five minutes can elevate the level by up to 15%
- Blood taken in the *evening* can give readings up to 15% higher
- Readings in *Winter* are around 5% higher than in *Summer*
- Strenuous *exercise* in the two to three hours before the sample is obtained may also alter the result
- Blood should be *dispatched promptly* to the laboratory or the readings will be altered.

Laboratory analysers may overestimate cholesterol levels by as much as 4%, and desktop analysers are even less accurate.[3]

A single cholesterol reading is not very useful. Repeated estimations will *regress to the norm* so that high readings will generally come down, and low readings will go up when repeated. It is suggested that treatment of cholesterol should be based on a minimum of two readings.[5] The Joint British Recommendations suggest the use of three readings, the first a random sample and (if abnormal) two more fasting samples.[16]

📄 **Guidelines**   **Taking a blood sample for cholesterol[5]**

The British Hyperlipidaemia Society has made the following recommendations

- Measurements are best performed in hospital chemical pathology departments
- Blood should be taken with minimum venous occlusion
- Subjects should have been sitting for 10 minutes before the test.

What to do with a cholesterol result

The level of serum cholesterol is only one of many risk factors for coronary events and coronary deaths. Successful prevention of heart attacks requires attention to all the alterable factors.

Is the cholesterol high? Take more than one reading: an individual may show variance up to 7% in their measured cholesterol.[3]

Is there an underlying disorder? Hypothyroidism, pregnancy, liver disease, diabetes and nephrotic syndrome can all raise cholesterol levels, as can excessive consumption of alcohol and caffeine.[17]

What are the other risks? Dealing with other risks will often be as productive as treating cholesterol levels.

📁 **Evidence**

Primary preventions of CHD[3]

Primary prevention NNTs for five years to avoid one coronary event for people at 3% a year CHD risk are:

Smoking advice		666
Nicotine replacement		333
Aspirin		333
Anti-hypertensive drugs for those	under 60	31
	over 60	26
Statins		21

📁 **Evidence**

Secondary preventions of CHD[3]

Secondary prevention NNTs for five years to avoid one coronary event for people at 3% a year CHD risk are:

Aspirin	37
Beta-blockers	30
Statins	26
Smoking advice	21
Oily fish	19
'Mediterranean' diet	19

These figures take into account the likely compliance with each intervention: for instance anti-smoking advice has a low chance of stopping people smoking, but smokers who have had a heart attack are more likely to stop than those who have not.

What does your patient want? If the CHD risk and cholesterol are high, some people are keener than others to take matters into their own hands by lifestyle alterations. Some will be happy to take tablets. Others will want to do nothing at all and accept their risk.

Treatment of raised cholesterol

For some patients it will be concluded, after assessment of their overall CHD risk, that artificially lowering the cholesterol will do some good. Treatment will *probably be lifelong*, so this is not a decision to be taken lightly. At the same time as cholesterol lowering is being considered, other risk factors should be addressed.

Smoking

Smoking is by far the *most important* avoidable risk factor for CHD. Cigarette smoking increases the risk of a heart attack roughly threefold (and more in younger people)[18] and doubles the risk in people who have had a heart attack and who continue to smoke.[19] Whatever else is done, every effort must be made to encourage patients to stop smoking. Among the many other cardiovascular risks of cigarette smoking, it also raises serum cholesterol slightly.

Diet

Diet is the mainstay of treatment for all types of hyperlipidaemia. There are two aims of dietary treatment

- Achieve ideal weight: a BMI of 25 kg/m^2 is desirable
- Reduce the amount of fat eaten, and alter the balance of fats in favour of the polyunsaturated variety.

Serum cholesterol is made largely from dietary fat, and to a much lesser extent from dietary cholesterol. *Polyunsaturated fats* tend to reduce serum cholesterol levels while saturated fats increase them.

The *Step One Diet* is recommended in the first instance. More rigid diets can be tried if this fails. The diet consists of

- Reducing *total fat* to less than 30% of calories
- Changing the *ratio* of polyunsaturated to saturated fats (the P:S ratio) to 1.0
- Total dietary *cholesterol* should be less than 300 mg a day
- *Calories* are reduced to achieve a desired weight.

In addition, *alcohol* intake will need to be within the recommended range (i.e. 21 units a week for a man and 14 units for a woman), or below this if obesity is a problem.

The improvement in cholesterol achievable by the adoption of the step one diet has been reported to be as high as 25%. However, such improvement is generally only possible when there is close dietary control. When free-living patients are looked at, the effect is less impressive, with a figure of 2% being more likely.[20] A very rigid diet will lower cholesterol levels substantially, but is very hard to keep to. A leaflet can be as effective as a chat with the practice nurse or with a dietician in reducing a patient's cholesterol through diet.[21] There is also concern that a cholesterol-lowering diet may reduce HDL more than total cholesterol, and so may adversely affect CHD risk.[22]

Dietary habits are not only a result of the choices which patients make. A diet which accords with the advice of the National Advisory Committee on Nutritional Education, a government-sponsored body, *costs around a third more* than a typical British diet.[23] Availability and palatability (which may well depend on tradition) are also influences.

Exercise

Regular moderate exercise reduces the risk of a heart attack by 60%.[24] In those who have already had a heart attack, exercise reduces the risk of recurrence by 25%.[25] In the previously sedentary, walking two miles in 30 minutes three times a week is sufficient,[25,26] and levels of activity can be subsequently built up.

Cholesterol-lowering drugs

Less than a third of people in England with a history of CHD or stroke are receiving lipid-lowering treatment, and of those on treatment less than a third have had their cholesterol lowered to the recommended level. An *inverse care law* probably applies: patients at lowest risk are more likely to seek treatment.[16]

The Joint British Recommendations suggest that if *total cholesterol* is unacceptably high, then it should be *reduced to 5.0 mmol/L* or below, and that *LDL cholesterol* should be *reduced to 3.0 mmol/L* or below.[9] Medication can be used if other methods of treatment have failed after a *trial of at least six months*.[5] Once drugs are started, treatment will usually be for life. As well as the costs and monitoring involved, there is also a psychological cost because of the creation of a 'patient'. The *dropout* rate from drug treatment will probably be around 20%,[27] but may be as high as 50%,[16] a concordance with medication rate significantly poorer than that achieved in the trials on which the benefits of drug treatment are based.

Statins or hydroxymethylgluterylcoenzyme-A reductase inhibitors are the latest, most powerful and the most expensive lipid-lowering agents available. They inhibit the liver pathways through which LDL is produced. They are highly effective with *reductions in cholesterol of up to 40%* and of triglycerides up to 20% being achievable. They are palatable and need to be taken only once a day. Side effects are few, a myositis with muscle pain occasionally developing. It is recommended that *liver function* be tested when a statin is being considered and measurements repeated periodically throughout treatment, and also that *creatine kinase* levels be checked regularly during treatment.[16] Most of the trials using statins have used simvastatin or pravastatin. The benefits seen are likely to be a *class effect*. Atorvastatin currently gives greatest cholesterol lowering when assessed by cost.[3] Cost effectiveness techniques have suggested that primary prevention with statins costs £136 000 and secondary prevention costs £32 000 per life-year saved (1996 prices).[28]

Anion exchange resins have been around for 20 years. They bind bile acids, making the liver produce more and using up cholesterol in the process. Cholesterol levels can by *reduced up to 20%*, but triglycerides may actually increase. The two currently available (cholestyramine and colestipol) are in granular form and need to be mixed with water. Gastrointestinal *side effects* such as bloating, flatulence and constipation are common, and mean that full compliance with treatment is unlikely.

Fibric acid derivatives are numerous and include bezafibrate, ciprofibrate and gemfibrozil. The parent, clofibrate, causes gallstones so is no longer used. They will reduce triglyceride levels up to 50%, and increase HDL levels up to 20%, but the *overall effect* on cholesterol is less predictable. Tolerance is usually good, with mild gastrointestinal symptoms being the only side effect.

Nicotinic acid in large doses reduces cholesterol and triglyceride by mechanisms not understood. It is hard to take because of *gastrointestinal side effects and flushing*. It is expensive at its higher recommended doses.

Starting drug treatment for raised cholesterol

If six months of effort with diet and exercise have failed to achieve the desired cholesterol levels, then patients of age 70 or under will benefit from drug treatment in primary prevention, and those of age 75 or under will benefit from secondary prevention.[29]

1. Ask about *alcohol and caffeine* consumption.
2. Check *blood* for diabetes, liver function, renal function and thyroid function all of which can elevate cholesterol.
3. *Prescribe* medication, which will be almost always a statin. Warn about muscle pain (possible myositis), and tell the patient to stop treatment if it occurs.
4. Urge *continuation of lifestyle measures*.
5. Review cholesterol level at *six to eight weeks*. The drug dose may need titrating. The doses of statins used in both the primary and secondary prevention trials tended to be large.
6. When and if the cholesterol falls to target continue drug treatment. Review level at least *once a year*. Check liver function and creatine kinase.
7. Patients established on drug treatment should *continue* even after they have reached the age when the evidence of benefit runs out.

The screening debate

In Britain an opportunistic programme for detecting raised cholesterol is advised but aimed only at those with a high risk of CHD. In America, using the same evidence, everyone is advised to have cholesterol levels checked during adult life.[5] Why should different conclusions have been reached? Arguments in favour of mass screening include:

- CHD is a very *important* cause of morbidity and mortality. Even a small reduction in risk will thus save a lot of illness and death
- The actual incidence of CHD is probably much higher than is known because of so-called *silent ischaemia* which is only apparent on electrocardiograph. As pre-existing CHD is a powerful reason for reducing

cholesterol, there is a lot of unmet need which will not emerge unless everyone is tested
- Case finding for *familial hyperlipidaemia* is at best 30% effective. Since this group have a lot to gain from treatment, up to 70% will be missed if screening is not routine.

Arguments for opportunistic screening include:

- In Britain nearly everyone is registered with a GP. Over 90% of the population visit their GP over a three-year period, so that *opportunistic screening* could detect the vast majority of cases of raised cholesterol
- Patients with an overall low CHD risk have *little to gain* from efforts to reduce their cholesterol. The chance finding of a raised level in someone who is otherwise well creates anxiety and may possibly lead to unnecessary treatment
- Patients with a normal cholesterol level but other risky habits may be *reassured* and so not motivated to alter. Even the finding of an abnormal cholesterol level is unlikely to motivate people to change their habits[15]
- The major known risk factors for CHD are the result of *personal habits* such as smoking, eating and exercise. These are only partly medical problems. Education and government policy will probably have as much impact as the one-to-one efforts of GPs.

Summary

- Raised serum cholesterol is an important risk factor for CHD. The higher the cholesterol, the greater the risk
- Raised serum cholesterol is one of many known risk factors for CHD, and the treatment of cholesterol should be based on the overall CHD risk
- Other modifiable risk factors for CHD are mainly matters of lifestyle and so less amenable to traditional medical intervention
- A single cholesterol measurement is of limited value
- At present it is wise to follow the Joint British Recommendations for the prevention of CHD. They are complicated and hard to use, and impossible to remember
- An annual CHD event risk of 3% is at present thought to be acceptable
- The statins have superseded nearly all other lipid-lowering agents. They are easy to take, cause a minimum of side effects, are highly effective, have been used in all the recent trials and cost a lot
- In Britain, opportunistic screening is recommended for cholesterol, population screening is not.

🗫 Topics for discussion

- Everyone should know their own cholesterol level
- The prevention of coronary heart disease is an individual responsibility
- The government target of reducing CHD events to 3% a year (1% a year CHD death) should be a subject for public debate
- Using the charts from the Joint British Recommendations (which can be found in the back of the British National Formulary) what is the CHD risk for a 53-year-old man being treated for hypertension, whose father died of a myocardial infarction when aged 54?

📖 **References**

1. Ball S, Betteridge J, Fairhurst G et al. Pocket guide to cholesterol 1995. London: Medical Imprint, 1995.
2. University of Leeds and University of York. Cardiac Rehabilitation. *Effective Health Care* 1998; 4(4): 1–12.
3. University of Leeds and University of York. Cholesterol and coronary heart disease: screening and treatment. *Effective Health Care* 1998; 4(1): 1–14.
4. Coronary heart disease: Statistics factsheet. London: British Heart Foundation, 1994.
5. Betteridge D J, Dodson P M, Durrington P N et al for the British Hyperlipidaemia Association. Management of hyperlipidaemia: Guidelines of the British Hyperlipidaemia Association. *Postgraduate Medical Journal* 1993; 69: 359–69.
6. Hyperlipidaemia: new evidence about treatment. *MeReC Bulletin* 1996; 7(4): 13–16.
7. Brown J G. Dietary control of blood cholesterol. Royal College of General Practitioners Members' Reference Book 1989. London: Sabrecrown Publishing, 1989, 319–20.
8. McGrath L T. How much faith can you place in a plasma lipid result? *Update* 1992; 45: 745–56.
9. British Cardiac Society, British Hyperlipidaemia Association, British Hypertension Society, British Diabetic Association. Joint British recommendations on prevention of coronary heart disease in clinical practice: summary. *BMJ* 2000; 320: 705–8.
10. Wallis J W, Ramsay L E, Ul Haq I et al. Coronary and cardiovascular risk estimation for primary prevention: validation of new Sheffield table in the 1995 Scottish health survey population. *BMJ* 2000; 320: 671–6.
11. Davey Smith G, Song F and Sheldon T A. Cholesterol lowering and mortality: the importance of considering initial level of risk. *BMJ* 1993; 306: 1367–73.
12. Shepherd J, Cobbe S M, Ford I et al for the West of Scotland Primary Prevention Study Group. Prevention of coronary heart disease with pravastatin in men with hypercholesterolaemia. *New Eng J Med* 1995; 333: 1301–7.
13. West of Scotland Coronary Prevention Group. West of Scotland Coronary Prevention Study: Identification of high-risk groups and comparison with other cardiovascular intervention tables. *Lancet* 1996; 348: 1339–42.
14. Robertson I, Phillips A, Mant D et al. Motivational effects of cholesterol measurement in general practice health checks. *Br J Gen Pract* 1992; 42: 469–72.
15. Scandinavian Simvastatin Survival Study group. Randomised trial of cholesterol lowering in 4444 patients with coronary heart disease: the Scandinavian Simvastatin Survival Trial (4S). *Lancet* 1994; 344: 1383–9.
16. Monkman D. Treating dyslipidaemia in primary care. *BMJ* 2000; 321: 1299–300.
17. Wierzbicki A. Hyperlipidaemia. *General Practitioner* April 1 1998: 62–4.
18. Parish S, Collins R, Peto R et al. Cigarette smoking, tar yields, and non-fatal myocardial infarction: 14 000 cases and 32 000 controls in the United Kingdom. *BMJ* 1995; 311: 471–7.
19. Thomson M. Post-MI care in general practice. *Update* 1998; 56: 636–45.
20. Ramsay L E, Yeo W W and Jackson P R. Dietary reduction of serum cholesterol concentration: time to think again. *BMJ* 1991; 303: 953–7.
21. Neil H A W, Roe L, Godlee R J P et al. Randomised trial of lipid lowering dietary advice in general practice: the effect on serum lipids, lipoproteins, and antioxidants. *BMJ* 1995; 310: 569–73.
22. Price D, Ramachandran S, Knight T et al. Observed changes in the lipid profile and calculated coronary risk in patients given dietary advice in primary care. *Br J Gen Pract* 2000; 50: 712–15.
23. Milne A. The cost of healthy eating. *Guardian* October 18 1986.

24. Brodie D. GPs should promote the benefits of exercise. *Monitor Weekly* 15 September 1993: 41–2.

25. Dargie H J and Grant S. Exercise. *BMJ* 1991; 303: 910–12.

26. Hardman A. Exercise and the heart: Report of the British Heart Foundation Working Group. London: BHF, 1993.

27. Andrade S E, Walker A M, Gottlieb L K et al. Discontinuation of anti-hyperlipidaemic drugs – do rates recorded in clinical trials reflect rates in primary care settings? *New Eng J Med* 1995; 332: 1125–31.

28. Pharaoh P D P and Hollingworth W. Cost effectiveness of lowering cholesterol concentration with statins in patients with and without pre-existing coronary heart disease: life table method applied to health authority population. *BMJ* 1996; 312: 1443–8.

29. Ritchie L D. Statins and the prevention of coronary heart disease: striking a balance that is desirable, affordable, and achievable. *Br J Gen Pract* 2000; 50: 693–4.

Dealing with dementia

Tutorial aims	**The registrar can make an initial assessment of a patient with dementia and plan their ongoing care in the community.**
Learning objectives	By the end of the tutorial the registrar can:

- List four types of dementia and give three clinical features of each
- Use a recognised tool to detect dementia
- Describe an initial physical assessment of a patient with dementia
- Describe the characteristics and needs of informal carers
- Help carers and sufferers plan ongoing care
- Discuss the ethical implications of impaired autonomy
- Discuss with a patient/carer the drawing up of an advance directive.

Preamble

It is estimated that in 1996 there were 678 000 people in the United Kingdom (UK) suffering from dementia, and that by 2021 this number will increase to 840 000.[1] Dementia is mainly a problem of *advancing age*, and so numbers of sufferers will increase as the numbers of the old and especially the very old rise.

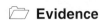 **Evidence**

The UK prevalence of dementia[2]	
40 to 65 years	1 per 1000
65 to 70 years	5 per 1000
70 to 80 years	20 per 1000
Over 80 years	200 per 1000

The average age of a patient suffering from dementia is 82, and there are four times as many *women* as men affected.[3] Around a third of sufferers at any one time are severely affected, and it is not known what proportion of those mildly affected will progress to severe dementia.[4] In primary care:

- A GP with a list size of 2000 will have approximately 22 patients with dementia, of whom between four and eight will require ongoing GP support[4]
- About 80% of patients with severe dementia, but only 30% of those with mild dementia, are known to their GP.[3]

Dementia care is costly. Taking into account hospital and residential care, GP care, day care, home care, and government payments made to informal carers, the total cost in 1995 was estimated at £1556 million.[5] This was more than the estimates for stroke (£949 million), diabetes (£748 million), and epilepsy (£156 million). In addition there is the contribution made by *informal carers*. In 1993 the Society of Actuaries estimated that each year care worth £30 billion was being provided by informal carers for the long-term sick and disabled in Britain.[6] The proportion of this consumed by the care of dementia is unknown, but it must be substantial. Cognitive impairment is the main reason for long-term institutional care.[7]

📁 **Evidence**

Costs of dementia care[8]	
In 1998 it was estimated that the weekly cost of caring for a patient with dementia was	
At home	£235
In a local authority institution	£390
In NHS hospital	£855

Recognising dementia

The early identification of dementia may reduce the risk of psychological illness in the carers, and the early mobilisation of support services may avert a crisis where the sufferer lives alone.[9]

In dementia there is cognitive impairment but a *normal level of arousal*. The presence of a normal conscious level distinguishes between dementia and toxic confusion. The cognitive deficit may at first be localised, often only affecting memory, and the patient may continue to function virtually normally. Later the cognitive impairment becomes more general, so fitting the formal criteria of dementia.

📄 **Guidelines**

Diagnostic criteria for dementia[10]

- Acquired deficit of cognition
- Multiple domains of cognitive impairment
- Must include memory impairment
- Cognitive impairment not due to disturbance of arousal
- Can be reversible

The two thirds of sufferers who are only mildly or moderately affected may well not be causing any great concern to their carers or medical advisers.

First Presentation

Typically the first indication of dementia is when the relatives or other *carers approach a GP* with their concerns. Such an approach will not have been made without a great deal of soul-searching and thought, and the carer must be given a sympathetic hearing. The recognition that a loved one's 'mind is going' is never easy, and neither is an admission by the carers that they are unable to cope. The *carers are rarely wrong* in their assessment, and their concerns should not be dismissed: establishing good relations at the outset leads to an improved therapeutic relationship, and the cooperation of the carers will be vital to the future care of the patient.

A patient with dementia may be quite unaware of their declining abilities, a phenomenon termed *anosognosia*. It is therefore essential to get a description from the carers about what is happening. Commonly problems will arise with respect to

- Difficulties at *work* (in those of working age) such as an unexpected dismissal
- A tendency to *mislay* items and forget appointments and names
- Failure to recognise people. Getting *lost* when out alone
- Recent changes in family role, for instance if someone suddenly stops taking responsibility for the family finances because of lack of memory.

Others are fully aware that their memory is deteriorating. When someone complains of declining memory, there is a good chance they are right. People who are in work of a demanding nature may be aware at an earlier stage of their declining powers.

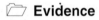 **Evidence**

Self-awareness of memory impairment[11]

In a population survey of people aged 65 to 85 who had not been diagnosed as either demented or depressed

- 34% reported that their memory was declining
- 37% were having daily living problems which could be attributed to poor memory.

Both these groups did less well on objective tests of cognitive function

---

In the more severely affected, memory complaints by patients correlate with depression, but memory complaints by relatives correlate with dementia.[12]

Presenting as a crisis   Dementia may cause crises because:

- There is commonly a *reluctance* to accept the diagnosis both by carers and sufferers. Only when the caring structure can cope no longer is a request made for help
- Many carers, particularly spouses, have a strong sense of *duty*, and want to take the burdens of care on themselves. They are usually elderly themselves, with declining powers, and as the patient's demands progress inexorably a breakdown occurs. The carer bears not only the accumulated effects of their caring, but also the sense of failure that they have not been able to cope

- If the main *carer* (the bulk of care usually falls to one person) *becomes ill* and cannot cope, then a crisis is likely
- Dementia is a *gradually worsening* condition, and so there is no obvious point at which a request for help is appropriate
- There may be a *new symptom* which is causing particular concern, such as wandering or night-time wakefulness
- Once a decision has been made to involve the GP, it is tempting for the carers to *justify* their decision with a detailed account of all the problems the dementia has caused, not just what has led to the current crisis
- Patients with dementia have reduced brain reserves and so are more likely to get *toxic confusion* if they contract an infection.

A GP faced with such a crisis may feel some resentment. In a gradually deteriorating situation earlier intervention might have averted the problem. It is, however, not fair to blame the carers for the crisis: they will often have been struggling with the problem for some time, and only turned to the GP as a last resort. Appropriate long-term care will often require a wide range of services, none of which can be set up straight away. It may be necessary to *admit* the patient to hospital if only to gain some time so that a proper management package can be organised.

Differential diagnosis

Dementia is a symptom, not a diagnosis. There are a number of types of dementia, and a number of other conditions which mimic dementia. Making a more detailed diagnosis than just 'dementia' is of practical importance since in some cases treatment is beneficial, and in some cases standard treatments are damaging.

Alzheimer's disease

Alzheimer's disease is named after Alois Alzheimer (1864 to 1915) who in 1906 first described the microscopic appearances in the brain. It is the *most common* cause of dementia in the UK with 400 000 sufferers, or around half of all those with dementia. In a further 20% of cases there is Alzheimer's disease as well as vascular dementia.[3] Alzheimer's disease is mainly a disease of old age, but 18 000 sufferers are below retiring age, and it is seen as early as the fourth decade.[13]

Alzheimer's disease is a histological diagnosis, confirmed only at post-mortem or biopsy. Clinicians, even specialists, are not very good at making the diagnosis based just on clinical assessment, *tending to over-diagnose* the illness.[14] In general this does not alter management except where a potentially remediable cause has been misdiagnosed as Alzheimer's.

In between 15 and 50% of cases there is thought to be an inherited predisposition for the illness,[15] and in up to *half of patients there is a family history*.[10] Homozygous possession of the apolipoprotein allele E-4 is associated with a tenfold increase in the risk of developing Alzheimer's disease.[3]

Alzheimer's disease is characterised by an *insidious onset and a gradual progression* of symptoms.[3] The most prominent cognitive deficit is of *memory*. Recent memory, such as recall for day-to-day events, deteriorates before memories accumulated from the past. Later there may be language problems and visuospacial difficulty. Frontal lobe features, such as loss of social skills, appear late. Delusions, hallucinations and aggression can occur, and these are particularly trying for the carers. Of the non-cognitive features, *depression* is the commonest and often occurs in the early stages of the disease.[10] Since depression can mimic dementia, in such cases it may be worth trying antidepressant treatment.

When a diagnosis of Alzheimer's disease has been made, the patient will usually be dead within four to ten years.[15]

Vascular dementia

Vascular dementia is less common than Alzheimer's disease, except in those over 85 in whom it may be commoner. It is the sole cause in about a third of patients with dementia, but a further third may have vascular dementia in addition to another cause.[16]

Vascular pathology may cause dementia in three ways

Multi-infarct dementia
Areas of the cortex and/or subcortical areas are damaged by small strokes. About 100 ml of brain tissue must be lost before symptoms of dementia become apparent.[16]

Single infarct dementia
The result of a larger stroke. Whether dementia occurs depends on the site of the stroke. A past stroke increases the risk of dementia ninefold.[16]

White matter dementia
Probably the commonest vascular dementia.[19] It was first described by Otto Biswanger in 1894, and so might be called Biswanger's disease. It can be the result of head injury or radiation damage, but is more commonly the result of ischaemia of the white matter. Around 10% of the elderly have CT evidence of white matter ischaemia, and this rises to 30% in those over 85.[16]

In the vascular dementias the intellectual deficit has a *sudden onset*, and then progresses in a *stepwise* manner,[3] as opposed to the gradual deterioration seen in Alzheimer's disease. Each worsening may be associated with transient *neurological loss* such as unsteadiness, or weakness of a limb. There may be a history of hypertension, old stroke or ischaemic heart disease. Clinical examination may reveal evidence of deteriorating vasculature.

Lewy body dementia

Lewy body dementia is increasingly recognised as a cause of dementia: at autopsy up to 20% of demented patients have Lewy bodies in their brain tissues.[17] Typically there are *fluctuating* levels of cognitive performance and frequent exacerbations of confusion. Visual hallucinations may occur. It is important to know if the dementia is of Lewy body type since the use of neuroleptic medication in this group is associated with increased mortality.[3]

The cause of the Lewy bodies is unknown. They occur in the cortex. In Parkinson's disease Lewy bodies are found in the substantia nigra: there is a tendency for Lewy body dementia and Parkinson's disease to co-exist.[3]

Frontal-type dementia

This constitutes around 10% of all dementias. There is a disturbance of *behaviour and personality* rather than memory. Speech deteriorates and may become repetitive, but *visuospacial skills* are preserved. In half of cases there is a family history of dementia.[3]

Rare dementias

This esoteric group constitutes about 5% of all dementias. Examples would be Pick's disease, Creutzfeld-Jakob disease and Huntington's chorea.

Depression

Depression occurs in around 3% of the over-65s, and another 10 to 15% will show some depressive symptoms.[18] In 25% of cases some cognitive impairment will result,[18] and occasionally this is bad enough to cause dementia-like symptoms, termed *pseudodementia*. On the other hand, depression is common among those with dementia. Dementing patients who are aware of their plight might be expected to feel depressed. All patients with dementia should be checked for depressive symptoms.

📂 **Evidence**

> **Prevalence of depression in Alzheimer's disease[19]**
>
> A study of 178 patients with a diagnosis of Alzheimer's disease found that:
>
> - 63% reported at least one depressive symptom
> - 43% were rated by carers as depressed
> - 24% were rated by a trained observer as depressed

The cognitive impairment in depression is a *problem of concentration* rather than of memory. The answers to the dementia questions are correct, it's just that the patient can't be bothered to take the test.

When diagnosing depression in the demented the same criteria apply as when making the diagnosis in the non-demented. The severity of symptoms and the presence of biological features will predict the success of antidepressant treatment. The choice of medication is influenced by the *presence of other health problems*: anticholinergic medication in patients with bladder outflow obstruction is to be avoided.

Toxic confusion

Toxic confusion is usually of *rapid onset*, and is also associated with *clouding of consciousness*, so it should not be too hard to distinguish from dementia. Patients who are already demented will have limited brain reserves and so are at increased risk of toxic confusion.

Age-associated memory impairment

This is a frequent though not universal finding among the elderly, especially those over 90 years. The brain shrinks to 80% of its maximum size by age 90. There is an episodic inability to remember names and dates. The information can be remembered at other times, however, which means that there is a problem with memory retrieval rather than with memory as such. This condition does not seem to get worse over time, and does not carry the mortality associated with Alzheimer's disease.[20]

**A practical approach
to diagnosis**

Most (up to 93%) of elderly people see their GP at least once in the course of a year, and those who do not rarely have health problems.[21] The offer to the over-75s of an annual check-up must include an assessment of mental well-being, including dementia.[22] Only a minority of persons with severe dementia are unknown to the caring services.

The problems posed by dementia are largely those of *care and management* rather than cure. The early identification of dementia allows more time for planning long-term care, and anticipates the needs not only of the patient but also of the carers.

The formal diagnostic criteria for dementia are ungainly when used in the practical situation. A number of ways round this have been devised using sets of standard questions. The one favoured by the Alzheimer's Disease Society is based on the Mental Status Questionnaire devised by Hodkinson.

📄 **Guidelines**

Testing for dementia[23]

For the 10 questions, 1 is scored for a correct answer, and 0 for a wrong answer

- What is your age? (Must be correct)
- What is the time? (To the nearest hour)
- Give the patient an address to recall at the end of the test (this must be a fictitious address, and the patient must be able to repeat it at the time to ensure that it has been heard correctly)
- What month are we in now? (Must be correct)
- What is the year now? (You can prompt with 'Two thousand and . . .'. Must be correct, except in January and February)
- What is the name of this place where we are now?
- What is your date of birth?
- What year did the First World War begin?
- Who is on the throne of England now?
- Please count backwards from 20 to 1, like this: 20, 19 . . . now you carry on
- Ask for the address given above. Number and street name should be correct

Scores:	8 to 10	normal
	7	probably abnormal
	6 and under	dementia confirmed

Between 10 and 15% of cases of dementia have a *treatable cause*: half of these patients have treatable intracerebral pathology, and half a systemic cause for the dementia.[18] A number of systemic diseases can cause a dementia-like illness. Commonest of these are anaemia and reduced perfusion causing cerebral anoxia. Other causes include heart failure, hypothyroidism, uraemia, vitamin B12 deficiency, alcohol abuse and occult carcinoma.

📄 **Guidelines**

GP investigations in dementia:[12]

- Urinalysis for protein and glucose

- Haemoglobin and full blood count and ESR for anaemia and B12 deficiency
- Thyroid stimulating hormone assay to check thyroid function
- Heart auscultation for evidence of heart failure, valve lesions or arrhythmia.

Any unexpected findings should prompt referral unless there is an easily remediable problem which can be treated in primary care. Situations which indicate that a CT scan might be helpful are:

- Clinical suggestion of raised intracranial pressure
- Focal neurological signs
- Recent head injury
- Evidence of cerebral infarction.

Managing dementia

Make the diagnosis

The carers will frequently have made the diagnosis before a doctor does. However it is important to confirm their impressions as the implications of the diagnosis are considerable, and the illness is terminal. If there is any doubt, the final verdict can be left to the specialist psychogeriatric or geriatric team. Whether the patient should be *told the diagnosis* is contentious. The newly available treatments for dementia need to be started in the early stages of the disease: if patients are not being told their diagnosis then consent to treatment cannot be truly informed, irrespective of the civil liberties issue of regarding all demented patients as mentally incompetent.

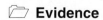 **Evidence**

> **Disclosure of diagnosis of dementia**
>
> - When a group of family members were asked whether their relative with Alzheimer's disease should be told their diagnosis, 83% said no. However, 71% of those same family members thought that they themselves should be told if they contracted the disease[24]
> - Only 44% of psychiatrists inform patients in the early stages of dementia[25]
> - Nearly half of GPs do not believe that making an early diagnosis of dementia does any good.[26]

Consider referral

All patients with suspected dementia should be referred for specialist assessment. Those suffering from mild or moderate Alzheimer's disease may benefit from drug treatment. In January 2001 the *National Institute for Clinical Excellence* issued a report on the drugs donepezil, rivastigmine and galantamine recommending that they be made available following specialist assessment and initiation to all patients who might benefit.[27] These drugs are all more effective in the early stages of dementia. More severe dementia gives rise to other management problems which may benefit from specialist assessment and inpatient care.

In most parts of the country a multidisciplinary *psychogeriatric team* is available and they are in the best position to make a full assessment. Referral gives the patient and carers the chance to get used to new professionals, and also ensures that any extra services can be arranged at the right time to avoid a crisis. If there has been referral to another medical professional, then there should also be a referral to a *social worker*. Advice on benefits is usually needed, and social services departments are the only way of accessing a number of supportive community services such as day care, home care, etc.

There is some evidence that carers of demented patients have incomplete *knowledge of available services*. In a survey from Dundee between a quarter and a third of carers were not aware of the community psychiatric nurse service, private domestic help, relatives' support groups, health visitors, geriatricians or hospital respite care.[28]

Support the carers

It is difficult to involve carers without having concerns about *confidentiality*. Carers need sufficient knowledge and understanding of the patient's disease to support their caring work, but this may mean that they end up being better informed than the patient. Proper assessment and treatment cannot be imposed unless the degree of the dementia is such that the patient is a danger to themselves or others.[29] Negotiating the path through these different constraints needs some careful footwork.

The key players in the care of the demented are the *informal carers*. To them falls the physical strain of their caring duties, which will often involve long hours and sheer hard work. A quarter of carers dedicate over 20 hours a week, and 15% spend up to 50 hours a week.[8] There is also the *emotional strain* of watching a loved one deteriorate intellectually so that they cease to be the person they were before. There will be loss of sociable conversation, continual questioning and demands for attention. Shouldering such a burden can only be described as heroic.

Respite care, day care or even permanent care may be required for the sake of the carer as much as the patient. Respite care delays institutionalisation, but does not help the carers feel any better.[12]

Advice about appropriate *benefits* will give a degree of financial confidence.

The GP can contribute by recognising the essential role of the carer in the team: carers should be regarded with the *same consideration and respect as other members of the primary healthcare team*. Requests to visit should be responded to promptly and without moaning. If a known carer attends the surgery, it is appropriate that they be seen with a minimum of delay to enable them to return to their caring duties.

Caring for people with dementia is stressful, and depression occurs in between 30 and 50% of carers.[30] The carers are just as likely to be depressed as the patient. It is particularly hard to find the physical and emotional resources to care for a demented relative if you are feeling depressed.

Behavioural problems are seen in around 70% of people with dementia.[31] The commonest presentations are agitation, aggression, wandering, shouting, disinhibition and sleep disturbance. Such symptoms are particularly difficult for carers to cope with, and are the single biggest factor leading to institutional care. Antipsychotics only help in around a quarter of cases.[31]

📄 **Guidelines**   **Dealing with behavioural problems**[31]

- Approach calmly
- Slow down and simplify
- Allow time to respond
- One-step commands
- Distraction
- Separate illness from person
- Humour can help

Self-help groups   The Alzheimer's Disease Society through its national organisation and 300 local groups provides support for carers and patients. Literature is produced for carers and patients, and also for professionals, to encourage the recognition and improve the management of patients with the disease.

> The Alzheimer's Disease Society
> Gordon House
> 10 Greencourt Place
> London SW1P 1PH
> Tel: 020 7306 0606

Unfortunately there is no evidence that carers' support groups reduce the stress of caring or alter outcome, even though they are generally perceived as being helpful.[12]

Medication   Restraints, be they chemical or physical, cannot ethically be used as a substitute for adequate staffing levels or a less rigid routine. Such restraint cannot, for example, be justified on the basis of reducing accidents since the evidence is that accidents are commoner in the restrained.[32] On the other hand dementia is commonly associated with challenging behaviour. Problems such as poor sleep and nocturnal wandering are particularly trying. In more severe cases there may be paranoia and violence, but usually by this stage the patient will be unable to remain in their own home.

Benzodiazepines tend to make cognitive impairment worse, even though they are very useful sedatives and are otherwise free of side effects. *Phenothiazines* cause sedation and Parkinson's-like movement disorders particularly in the elderly. Postural hypotension may be a problem, and there are important interactions with some antidepressants and antiepileptics. Neuroleptics should not be used in patients with *Lewy body dementia*. Thioridazine used to be the most widely used as the side effects were less, but this has now been prevented by concerns over cardiotoxicity. The new antipsychotic risperidone is now probably the drug of choice.[31]

On microscopic and biochemical analysis, the brains of patients who have died from *Alzheimer's disease* are different from normal brains. These differences have in turn suggested drug treatments specific for the disease. Tacrine is licensed in the United States, and an increasing number of *acetylcholinesterase inhibitors* (e.g. donepezil) are available in the UK for the symptomatic treatment of mild to moderate Alzheimer's disease. At best these agents slow the decline in Alzheimer's sufferers rather than reverse the disease process.

There is no specific treatment for *vascular dementia*, but low dose aspirin should be considered in those not already taking it. Treatment of other vascular pathology, especially atrial fibrillation, may be of value.

Enduring power of attorney (EPA)

A person who becomes demented may wish to appoint someone to run their affairs against the time when they are unable to do so for themselves. This is done by setting up an EPA.

The deed setting up the EPA must be *signed by both parties and the signatures witnessed* (but not necessarily by a doctor or lawyer) at a time when the patient is *still capable* of giving agreement. The attorney is not allowed to gain by their ministry of the affairs, and if found to do so the control reverts to the Court of Protection for the appointment of a receiver.

Testamentary capacity

A GP may be asked to decide whether or not a patient has the ability to make a valid will. To do so the patient has to be able to appreciate what the *value* of their estate is, and *who may have claims* on the estate. At this stage the wise GP will at least consider referral to a specialist colleague.

Driving

Patients with mild dementia may still drive. Since much mild dementia is unknown to doctors and is not recognised by the sufferers, it can be assumed that many patients with mild dementia are in fact driving. Advancing cognitive impairment makes driving unsafe, as does any degree of visuospacial impairment. The presence of dementia *should be reported* to the DVLA. Family members will usually be in agreement with this as many fear for their safety when being driven. If the patient with dementia will not report their diagnosis, the GP has a professional duty to notify the DVLA if a patient is driving while unfit.

Advance directive (living will)

An advance directive is a means by which a person can extend their control over the types of medical treatment they want to a time when they are mentally incapable of making decisions contemporaneously.

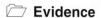 **Evidence**

> **Deciding to die**
>
> - It is estimated that at some time 70% of Americans will have to decide, or have decided on their behalf, whether or not to continue supportive medical intervention during an incurable disease process.[33]
> - In Britain 86% of elderly people would not want artificial ventilation if they were too confused to be safely left alone, and 90% would not wish cardiopulmonary resuscitation if they were so senile that they were unable to recognise family and friends.[34]

The right of a mentally competent person to refuse treatment is well established in English common law. The first Advance Directive was suggested by Luis

Kutner, a Chicago lawyer, in 1969. A House of Lords Select Committee considered the issue in 1994 and concluded that specific legislation in Britain was not necessary. The Crown Prosecution Service, the Law Commission and the British government have all endorsed the view that an advance directive is *legally binding*, and this has also been reinforced by High Court ruling.[34]

Any GP who is aware of the existence and content of an advance directive but fails to comply with it may be held *guilty of assault*. Conversely the withholding of treatments at the specific request of an advance directive is not culpable. GPs cannot be forced by an advance directive to do (or not do) something against which they hold a moral objection. In such circumstances the GP is professionally bound to *hand on the care* of the patient to another practitioner who will comply with the directive.

An advance directive is only valid in so far as it specifies treatments which the patient refuses: it cannot be used as a demand for specific treatments. It cannot be used as a request for assisted death or anything else which is currently illegal.

An advance directive should only be made *after taking medical advice*. The GP may therefore have quite an involved role. The idea of an advance directive should be discussed and then the document drawn up; the GP will need some system of knowing which patients have drawn up an advance directive; the advance directive will need periodic review; and its provisions will have to be complied with.

The content of an advance directive needs to cover several issues, for instance which treatments are being refused, and in which medical circumstances the directive is to be used. A patient contemplating the drawing up of an advance directive is best advised to obtain one of the model texts published by Age Concern, the Centre of Medical Law and Ethics or the Voluntary Euthanasia Society.

Instead of signing an advance directive, some patients may wish to appoint a trusted friend or relative to make health decisions on their behalf should they become mentally incompetent to do so themselves. In English law, *power of attorney* only applies to the estate, but there are proposals before parliament to allow a patients to appoint a proxy to make healthcare decisions on their behalf at such time as they are mentally not competent to do so for themselves.[34]

Consent to treatment

The presence of dementia may limit a person's ability to make choices, but only in extreme cases is that ability completely destroyed. Most dementia sufferers have at least *partial autonomy*. All adults have the right to make choices for themselves, however wrong those choices may appear to others. An adult has legal capacity to give or refuse consent to medical treatment if he or she can[35]

- Understand and retain the information relevant to the decision in question
- Believe that information
- Weigh that information in the balance to arrive at a choice.

Summary

- Dementia is a problem of older people, and so will probably become more common in the future
- Dementia is a symptom, not a diagnosis. Different causes of dementia may require different management. A minority of dementia is curable
- Many patients with dementia get depressed, and some of the depressed develop cognitive impairment
- Support for carers is one of the more important management priorities. Carers may be working up to 50 hours a week on their duties, and are as likely to become as depressed as the patient. Carers should be afforded appropriate respect as key members of the primary care dementia team
- Newer treatments for Alzheimer's disease should be initiated only from secondary care
- An advance directive, indicating the types of treatment which a patient wishes to refuse, is legally binding in the UK.

Topics for discussion

- All sufferers from dementia should be encouraged at an early stage to draw up an advance directive
- Correcting the 'post-code rationing' of treatment for Alzheimer's disease is a public health priority
- The national economy is likely to collapse under the burden of caring for dementia
- The worst people to look after patients with dementia are family members
- Dementia is indicative of a terminal disease process. Accurate diagnosis and early disclosure are as important in dementia as they are in any other terminal disease.

References

1. Opening the mind: new frontiers in Alzheimer's research. London: Alzheimer's Disease Society, 1996.
2. Fairburn A F. Alzheimer's disease and its management. *Prescribers Journal* 2000; 40(2): 77–85.
3. Coates T. Dementia. *General Practitioner* March 1 1996: 55–9.
4. Philp I. Challenges of dementia to the GP: five areas to attack. *Geriatric Medicine* 1989; 19(11): 19–20.
5. Gray A M. The costs of Alzheimer's disease. Geriatric Medicine 1996; 26(9), suppl: 3.
6. Tonks A. Community care fails the frail and elderly. *BMJ* 1993; 307: 1163.
7. Melzer D, Ely M and Brayne C. Cognitive impairment in elderly people: population based estimate of the future in England, Scotland and Wales. *BMJ* 1997; 315: 462.
8. Bosanquet N. Alzheimer's disease. *Geriatric Medicine* 1999; 29(4): 13–14.
9. O'Neill K. Dementia: a practical approach. *Update* 1999; 58: 33–9.
10. Rosser M. Alzheimer's Disease. *BMJ* 1993; 307: 779–82.
11. McIntosh I. One-third of older people have memory problems. *Medical Monitor* 3 April 1996: 38.
12. North of England Evidence Based Dementia Guideline Development Group. North of England evidence based guidelines development project: guideline for the primary care management of dementia. *BMJ* 1998; 317: 802–8.
13. Gray A. and Fenn P. Alzheimer's Disease: the burden of the illness in England. *Health Trends* 1993; 25: 31–7.

14. Homer A C, Honavar M, Lantos P L et al. Diagnosing dementia: Do we get it right? *BMJ* 1988; 297: 894.
15. Kennedy A. Alzheimer's. *General Practitioner* October 15 1993: 35–42.
16. Amar K and Wilcock G. Vascular dementia. *BMJ* 1996; 312: 227–31.
17. McConville P and Whalley L J. Confusion and dementia. *Update* 1997; 54: 765–74.
18. Nalpas A. I think my wife's memory is slipping, doctor. *Monitor Weekly* 1993; 6(41): 44–7.
19. Burns A, Jacoby R and Levy R. Psychiatric phenomena in Alzheimer's disease. III: Disorders of mood. *Br J Psychiatry* 1990; 157: 81–6.
20. O'Brien J T and Levy R. Age associated memory impairment. *BMJ* 1992; 304: 5–6.
21. Perkins E R. Screening elderly people: a review of the literature in the light of the new general practitioner contract. *Br J Gen Pract* 1991; 41: 382–5.
22. Terms of Service for Doctors in General Practice. London: DoH, 1989.
23. Hodkinson H M. Evaluation of a mental test score for assessment of mental impairment in the elderly. *Age Ageing* 1972; 1: 233–8.
24. Maguire C P, Kirby M, Coen R et al. Family members' attitudes towards telling the patient with Alzheimer's disease their diagnosis. *BMJ* 1996; 313: 529–30.
25. McIntosh I. Ethical issues in AD. *Geriatric Medicine* 1999; 29 No 9: 4–5.
26. Renshaw J, Scurfield P, Cloke L and Orrell M. General practitioners' views on the early diagnosis of dementia. *Br J Gen Pract* 2001; 51: 37–8.
27. National Institute for Clinical Excellence. Guidance on the Use of Donepezil, Rivastigmine and Galantamine for the treatment of Alzheimer's Disease. London: DoH, 2001.
28. Philp I, McKee K J, Meldrum P et al. Community care for demented and non-demented elderly people: a comparison study of financial burden, service use, and unmet needs in family supporters. *BMJ* 1995; 310: 1503–6.
29. Matthews K and Milne S. How and when to apply the Mental Health Act. *The Practitioner* 1994; 238: 398–404.
30. Ballard C G, Eastwood C, Gahir M et al. A follow up of depression in the carers of dementia sufferers. *BMJ* 1996; 312: 947.
31. Baldwin A C and Rigby J C. Dementia: Management of behavioural problems. *Geriatric Medicine* 2001; 31(4): 61–4.
32. Walsh K and Bennett G. Restraint. *Geriatric Medicine* 2000; 30(11): 24–7.
33. McLean S A M. Making Advance Medical Decisions. *Journal of the Medical and Dental Defence Unions* 1995; 12(2): 28–9.
34. Dyer C. Power of attorney change in England and Wales. *BMJ* 1999; 319: 211.
35. Halstead G A and Vernon M J. Are you confused about consent? *Geriatric Medicine* July 2000: 19–23.

Diabetes

<table>
<tr><td>

Tutorial aim

</td><td>

The registrar can manage diabetes appropriately in primary care.

</td></tr>
<tr><td>

Learning objectives

</td><td>

By the end of the tutorial the registrar can:

- List five possible presentations of diabetes
- Recall five complications of diabetes
- Give four reasons for referral to hospital
- Discuss the importance of controlling blood sugar and blood pressure
- Discuss the importance of a diabetic diet
- Describe the involvement of the team in primary care diabetic management
- Help a diabetic choose suitable treatment.

</td></tr>
</table>

Introduction

In either the second or third century, Aretaeus the Cappadocian described diabetes thus:

> "Diabetes is a wonderful affection, not very frequent among men, being a melting down of the flesh and limbs into urine. The course is a common one, namely, the kidneys and the bladder; for the patients never stop making water, but the flow is incessant, as if from the opening of aqueducts. The nature of the disease is long-lived, but the patient is short-lived. Moreover, life is disgusting and painful; thirst unquenchable; excessive drinking which, however, is disproportionate to the large quantity of urine. One cannot stop them from drinking or making water"

About 2% of the population of the UK have diabetes,[1] two thirds of which is diagnosed.[2] A GP will on average deal with two or three new diabetics each year, and will have a further 20 to 30 already diagnosed cases on the list.[2]

Type 1 diabetes

Previously 'insulin-dependent' or IDDM. Characterised by a failure of insulin production.

- The annual incidence of new cases in the age range 0 to 15 is about 20 per 100 000. Most present at age 9 to 13, but a quarter are diagnosed under the age of five[3]
- The incidence of new cases has increased markedly in Europe, typically by 50% in the last 30 years.[4]

Type 2 diabetes
Previously 'non-insulin dependent' or NIDDM. A problem of older people, characterised by insulin resistance in the tissues. Levels of circulating insulin may be greater than normal, but there is invariably also some failure of insulin production before diabetes becomes clinically apparent.[5]

- The prevalence of Type 2 diabetes is about 200 per 100 000,[5] and this has risen by up to 50% in the last 20 years probably due to the increased prevalence of obesity[6]
- The incidence and prevalence of Type 2 diabetes rises with age, and is slightly greater in women
- Over 60 years of age about 3% of people have diabetes, and this rises to 4% in the over-70s[2]
- Among Asian immigrants to the UK the prevalence is much higher, at 10% overall and 16% in the over-65s.[7]

The risks of diabetes
Diabetics have more than *three times the mortality* of non-diabetics,[2] and cost the NHS £2 billion a year[8] (2000 prices). The health risks of diabetes are nearly all mediated through small blood vessel (microvascular) and large blood vessel (macrovascular) complications: fluctuations in blood sugar levels may cause the occasional acute illness, but it is the vascular complications which kill and maim.

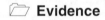 **Evidence**

Extra morbidity in diabetics[9]	
Compared with the non-diabetic population, diabetics bear additional morbidity risks of:	
Blindness	20 times risk
End-stage renal disease	25 times risk
Amputation	40 times risk
Myocardial infarction	2 to 5 times risk
Stroke	2 to 3 times risk

Diabetic eye disease
- Nearly 10% of diabetics are *registered blind*,[2] and half of these will be dead inside four years with only one in five surviving more than 10 years[10]
- Eye complications in diabetes are caused by microvascular pathology. A fifth of Type 2 diabetics have retinopathy when diagnosed[9]
- After 10 years, 10% of patients with Type 1 and 50% of those with Type 2 diabetes will have retinopathy, and after 25 years 90% of all diabetics will be affected.[10]

Non-proliferative (background) retinopathy Abnormal arterial wall permeability leads to the fundoscopic findings of *haemorrhages, exudates and oedema*. It is commonest in Type 2 diabetics. Only 3% of patients with background retinopathy will have any visual impairment after five years, so the prognosis is excellent.

Proliferative retinopathy In addition to background retinopathy there is optic disc and peripheral retinal *neovascularisation* (new vessel formation) and vitreous haemorrhage. Retinal ischaemia is thought to give rise to these effects. Proliferative retinopathy is virtually unknown in patients with diabetes of under five years' duration, and only rare under 10 years. However, at 30 years, 60% of Type 1 diabetics will have developed the disorder, a much higher proportion than in Type 2 where only 30% ever develop it.[11] Proliferative retinopathy is sight-threatening, but in 80% of cases the sight can be saved by using the argon laser.[11]

Diabetic maculopathy: is diagnosed when there are *microaneurysms* clustered near the macula, *macular oedema, hard exudates and haemorrhages*. This is also due to ischaemia, and affects Type 2 (30%) more than Type 1 diabetics (10%) patients. This too is potentially sight-threatening, but in 60% of cases the argon laser will save the sight.[11]

Detecting Retinopathy Hospital consultants, ophthalmic opticians and specially interested and trained GPs seem to be *equally proficient* at detecting retinopathy,[11] and all are rather better than the untrained GP. In a number of areas the health authority will finance opticians to provide an annual free eye check to confirmed diabetics. Fundoscopy through undilated pupils, whoever does it, will miss between a third and two thirds of cases of retinopathy.[12] As diabetics with retinopathy are also more likely to have neuropathy, their pupils are often abnormally small making the view even more restricted. A combination of fundoscopy and retinal photography, both through *dilated pupils*, appears to be the best way of detecting pathology.[12]

Nephropathy

Among diagnosed diabetics 15% have proteinuria, and if they live long enough 75% will develop renal failure.[2] Microalbuminuria, that is proteinuria too slight to show up on an Albustix, is a marker for a high risk of progression to frank nephropathy. Perfect control of blood pressure will prevent renal failure.[13]

Neuropathy

Sensory neuropathy affects half of diabetics.[9] Half of diabetic men have erectile dysfunction, and 25% of diabetics are at risk of foot disease.[2] The combination of neuropathy with poor circulation may lead to persistent lesions which can only be dealt with by amputation.

Arteriosclerosis

The diabetic complications considered so far are the result of microvascular involvement. However, in terms of mortality the macrovascular complications are much more important: about 75% of diabetics will eventually die of an arteriosclerotic cause[14] (heart attack, stroke), and 3% have intermittent claudication.[2]

- Known cardiovascular risk factors tend to cluster in diabetics: hypertension, obesity, raised cholesterol and lack of exercise
- Diabetics are just as likely to smoke as anyone[15]
- In addition, the diabetes confers an extra independent risk so that for any given risk factor the diabetic will run between two and four times the

cardiovascular risk of the non-diabetic.[16] This extra risk may be the result of diabetic cardiomyopathy.[17]

- If they have a heart attack, diabetics are twice as likely to die.[9]

Diagnosing diabetes

Type 1 diabetes usually presents relatively *acutely* in a young patient. There is *thirst, polyuria and weight loss* over the course of two or three weeks.[3] In the younger child these symptoms are more difficult to identify, and so the presentation may be of vague ill health, and eventually breathing difficulties due to acidosis. Severe *abdominal pains* can be brought on by ketoacidosis. In some cases the disease is more rapid and the child becomes unwell over a few hours with profound *dehydration*.

Type 2 diabetes presents more gradually, and has commonly existed for *10 to 12 years before diagnosis.*[18] Glycosuria may be found on routine testing of the asymptomatic. On direct questioning, however, it is usual to elicit some symptoms. Sometimes there is the classical picture of thirst, polyuria and weight loss. Other presentations include tiredness, pruritis vulvae, blurred vision (the osmotic effect of the increased glucose in the lens causes swelling), foot ulceration, balanitis or recurrent sepsis. There may be the effects of arteriosclerosis such as intermittent claudication, myocardial infarction or stroke.

Testing the urine for glucose is a routine part of the new patient medical, the well person check and the antenatal clinic attendance. Curiously, looking for glycosuria is not a mandatory part of the over-75 check.

Urine testing is the simplest way of estimating blood sugar levels, but it only gives an approximate measure. In people with a low renal threshold, for example, it is possible to find glycosuria in the presence of a normal blood sugar. If this is the case, there is no diabetes, but other aspects of renal functioning should be investigated. The renal threshold can increase with age.[14]

📄 Guidelines

Confirming diabetes:[19]

The World Health Organisation and the British and American Diabetic Associations now endorse the views of the American Expert Committee Report of 1997. Diabetes is confirmed where:

- Symptoms of diabetes and random plasma glucose ≥ 11.1 mmol/L
- Fasting (eight hours with no calories) plasma glucose ≥ 7.0 mmol/L
- Plasma glucose ≥ 11.1 mmol/L two hours after 75 g oral glucose.

Aims of treatment

The risks of diabetes have to be minimised, but not at the expense of making life intolerable.

Minimise symptoms

If blood sugar is too high or too low then symptoms result. Hypoglycaemia causes greater problems because it tends to come on suddenly. Diabetes is frequently diagnosed at a stage when symptoms are not particularly severe: it would be unreasonable to substitute this for a treatment which actually makes the patient feel worse.

Attempt normoglycaemia

Keeping blood sugars as near the normal range as possible reduces microvascular complications in Type 1[20] and in Type 2[21] diabetes. However, tighter blood glucose results in greater weight gain and more episodes of hypoglycaemia,[22] even though the hypoglycaemia is well tolerated.[23] There is a *continuous relationship* between glycaemic control and microvascular complications, so it is not clear what the target blood sugar should be.[9]

📄 **Guidelines**   **Blood sugar targets in diabetic care[24]**

The British Diabetic Association (BDA) recommends:

- HbA1c ≤7.0%
- Fasting blood glucose of 4 to 7 mmol/L
- Self-monitored blood glucose before meals of 4 to 7 mmol/L

Control blood pressure

Around 40% of diabetics also have raised blood pressure.[25] There is a *linear relationship* between the level of blood pressure and the cardiovascular risk, so that there is no obvious target.[26] Reducing the pressure significantly reduces microvascular complications, diabetes-related deaths and stroke, but not myocardial infarction or all-cause death.[25] Which medication is used to reduce blood pressure does not seem to matter,[25] and at least a third of diabetics will need three or more drugs to achieve satisfactory control.[9] Angiotensin-converting enzyme (ACE) inhibitors may protect against neuropathy and retinopathy independently of any blood pressure reduction, and so are probably first choice agents for diabetics.[9]

📄 **Guidelines**   **Blood pressure target in diabetes[24]**

Without macrovascular complications	140/80
With macrovascular complications	130/80
With proteinuria	125/75[27]

Minimise complications

Regular monitoring of feet, nerves, kidneys and eyes will ensure that the best treatment is secured if complications do occur.

Reduce the risk of cardiovascular disease

As so many diabetics die of cardiovascular disease, reducing this risk is of major importance. Diabetes is an extra risk factor which has to be taken into account when assessing overall risk. For instance, the Joint British recommendations on the prevention of coronary heart disease suggest that the target cholesterol level for diabetics should be the same as for patients who already have CHD.[27]

The newly diagnosed diabetic

Some new diabetics will present acutely unwell with ketoacidosis and require immediate hospital admission. These are usually the younger patients who have Type 1 diabetes. The symptoms in the more common Type 2 diabetes are generally much less dramatic, and so management can be undertaken in primary care.

The first consultation

With a newly diagnosed diabetic this should seek to answer the following questions:

- Is the diabetes *secondary* to another pathology such as pancreatic failure, or secondary to steroid therapy?
- Is there any evidence of microvascular or macrovascular *complications*? Any found will usually require referral for further assessment
- What is the overall *cardiovascular risk*, and can anything be done to reduce it?

History

Details of drugs, symptoms of cardiovascular disease.

Examination

Weight, height, blood pressure, visual acuity, fundi.

Tests

Glucose and either glycosylated haemoglobin (HbA1c) or fructosamine (if not already done in the course of making the diagnosis), urea and electrolytes, lipid profile.[28] Measuring HbA1c is expensive, and readings are affected by haemoglobinopathies, uraemia and alcoholism. The reading obtained represents an average of glucose levels *over the previous three months*, which may mask wide fluctuations. Fructosamine gives an indication of blood glucose levels over a much shorter time, but is cheaper to do.[29]

Patient information

Some patients already suspect that they are diabetic, and so will have already begun the mental adjustment process. Others will react with disbelief or even frank denial. Yet others will react with anger or regard the diagnosis as a sentence of imminent and painful death. A loss reaction is occurring: loss of health and loss of an expected future. Cooperation with treatment is important. Having diabetes has *lifelong implications*. Better glycaemic control is more likely when the patient has sufficient *knowledge* of their diabetes.[30] Sharing information is not just a matter of common courtesy, it also influences long-term physical health.

The BDA publishes excellent self-help material for diabetics.

British Diabetic Association,
10 Queen Anne Street
London W1M 0BD
Tel: 020 7323 1531

The diabetic diet

Whatever other therapy is used, a suitable diet should also be advised. Access to the services of a *dietician is essential* to optimise management.[29] For diabetics who are to be managed in primary care, if a community dietetic service does not exist (as it does not in many areas), then referral to the local hospital department is needed.

A diet should be *tailored to individual needs and tastes*. The aim of a diabetic diet is that sugars from the food are released into the blood gradually. Even highly complex and sophisticated regimens of insulin injection cannot hope to match the efficiency with which the normally functioning pancreas reacts to fluctuating blood sugar levels. The hypoglycaemic therapies available bring about an even rate of removal of sugar from the blood, and this should be matched by an even rate of the appearance of sugar in the blood if wide fluctuations in blood sugar level are to be avoided.

- To achieve this the diet should contain 50 to 60% of its calories in complex carbohydrates, while simple sugars are restricted. Fibre content should be high as this slows the absorption of the sugars from the gut[29]
- Three quarters of people with newly diagnosed Type 2 diabetes are obese[31] The overweight will need some calorie restriction in order to reduce the body mass index to 25 kg/m^2 or under for preference, and certainly under 27 kg/m^2. A low-fat diet is a good general principle, and those with elevated lipid levels will need special attention in this respect[29]
- Diabetics who do shift work, heavy manual jobs or who are involved in sport will require special attention from the dietetics team.

Oral hypoglycaemic medication

Under one in five of those who have Type 2 diabetes will be controlled at three months by diet alone.[32]

Biguanides

Metformin is the only biguanide drug available in the United Kingdom. It works by reducing glucose absorption from the gut, and by increasing insulin sensitivity.[5] It is the only diabetic treatment which reduces the amount of circulating insulin (with the consequent theoretical reduction in cardiovascular risk), and does not cause weight gain. It does not cause hypoglycaemic episodes. It is first choice treatment in the overweight diabetic.[25] The starting dosage is 500 mg twice a day, rising to a maximum of 2 g or even 3 g a day if tolerated. The commonest side effects are gastro-intestinal, and in particular *diarrhoea* (which is consistent with its mode of action). Metformin should not be used in severe heart failure, renal or hepatic failure, or in heavy users of alcohol because of the risk of lactic acidosis: this only occurs in one to eight cases per 100 000 patient-years, but carries a mortality of up to 50%.[33]

Sulphonylureas

Sulphonylureas work by boosting the insulin output of the pancreas, and so will only be effective where there is some residual beta cell activity. In long-term use there are also some extra-pancreatic actions. They are first choice treatment in diabetics of normal weight.[25] Members of this class of drugs are about equally effective, but there are differences in their duration of action.

- The longer-acting *chlorpropamide* and *glibenclamide* can cause prolonged and profound hypoglycaemia which is particularly problematic in the elderly

- *Tolbutamide* is cheap, short-acting, and has a proven track record of safety, but has to be taken up to three times a day
- *Gliclazide* is more expensive, but can be used once a day and can be used if there is renal impairment, as it is inactivated in the liver.

All sulphonylureas may cause rashes and weight gain. Trimethoprim, sulphonamides and the 4-hydroxyquinolones may increase their effect, as may miconazole and possibly fluconazole. There is a possible toxic interaction with ketotifen. Use with metformin is synergistic.

Acarbose

Acarbose is an alpha glucosidase inhibitor which reduces blood sugar when used together with diet alone, or with other hypoglycaemics. It can cause flatulence and diarrhoea, and its effects may decrease with time. It has yet to establish its place in diabetes treatment.[25]

Glitazones

This is the newest group of oral hypoglycaemics available in Britain. The National Institute for Clinical Excellence has suggested the use of rosiglitazone or pioglitazone in combination with either a sulphonylurea or metformin when a combination of these latter two is unsuccessful. When using a glitazone additional monitoring with periodic liver function tests is needed.[34]

Choice of Medication

Drug treatment should only be considered if three months of dietary treatment have not secured normoglycaemia and symptomatic improvement.

The *overweight* are best started on metformin, and the rest on a sulphonylurea. Treatment should be increased monthly up to the maximum if the blood sugars are still high. If after three months at maximum treatment blood sugar is not controlled, or before if the patient still feels unwell, then either a combination of metformin and a sulphonylurea can be used, or consideration given to insulin treatment.

📄 Guidelines

Reasons to start insulin:[5]

- Inadequate control with diet, exercise and maximal oral agents, especially if associated with unintentional weight loss
- Intercurrent events such as severe infections, surgery or myocardial infarction
- Renal impairment
- Diabetic complication.

Insulin

The establishment of an insulin regime is, in my view, a job for a specialist. A written, individualised programme should be available of how and when the insulin dose should be altered. This will be informed by regular if infrequent blood sugar assessments: it is usually more useful to obtain several readings on one day rather than to get one reading at the same time every day. The role of the GP is in monitoring and helping with the interpretation of the programme. GPs with a special interest and expertise may wish to become involved in the modification of the insulin programme, but not to the exclusion of specialist input either through the hospital clinic or through the specialist community diabetic nurse.

Intercurrent illness If an intercurrent illness occurs, the so-called 'sick days' in diabeticspeak, blood sugar will tend to rise. Insulin (if used) or oral hypoglycaemics should not be stopped,[29] whatever eating pattern the intercurrent sickness enforces. If the sugars rise excessively, or if the patient is showing signs of ketoacidosis and especially if this produces vomiting of more than a few hours duration, then admission to hospital is required.

Follow-up of a diabetic[9]

At least *once a year* there should be an extensive check-up, with lesser reviews every four to six months.

Narrative

- Ask about *symptoms* including details of any hypoglycaemic episodes, time off work or school, episodes of nocturnal frequency and the development of erectile dysfunction
- Cigarette smoking. Calculate and discuss *cardiovascular* risk
- Treatment review with reference to blood sugars
- Check *understanding* of diabetes, diet and medication
- Is input from chiropody, dietetics or the specialist diabetic nurse needed?

Clinical examination

- Weight
- Visual acuity for near and distance vision
- Fundoscopy with dilated pupils
- Blood pressure
- Peripheral pulses
- Foot sensation, vibration sense, ankle reflexes.

Biochemical

- Blood should be taken for:[29]

  glucose
  either HbA1c or fructosamine
  serum creatinine
  blood lipids

Microalbuminuria should be checked for as this predicts later renal problems.

Nearly all diabetics *cheat on their diet* and about a fifth do so every day.[35] It is important to ask direct questions in order to get at the truth. Dietary lapses may be the consequence of incomplete understanding or the unsuitability of the diet: in such cases further assessment and education are required. Some diabetics, especially the adolescents, will deliberately alter their diet to produce episodes of hypo- or hyper-glycaemia. This phenomenon must be viewed in the light of the overall family dynamics if it is to be understood and managed. Happily the problem is usually self-limiting without too much damage being done.

Diabetic education should observe a number of educational ground rules:[29]

- Aims and objectives should be defined and agreed
- The programme should be tailored to the patient, not vice versa
- Not too much information should be offered at one time
- Essentials should be dealt with first
- Teaching should occur at appropriate times and in appropriate settings: sometimes small group sessions are effective. Literature and experienced patients can be valuable resources
- All members of the care team should have a consistent approach to diabetes.

Only a minority of diabetics monitor their blood sugars properly, but those that do achieve better glycaemic control.[36]

What do diabetics want?

The above routine of checks is broadly in agreement with the recommendations of the BDA.[37] Most diabetics want as much information as possible about their illness and its implications. In addition to the medical aspects of care, information will be needed about work, driving, insurance and prescription charges. Regular physical check-ups are valued as is input from professional health workers, especially a dietician. There is also a need to be able to contact a member of the healthcare team for advice when necessary.

Is primary or secondary care best?

In the past it was normal for all diabetics to be followed up by the hospital services. This is unnecessary, inconvenient for the patients, and puts an unreasonable strain on the hospital clinics. In any case it is often the most junior doctors who staff hospital diabetic clinics, doctors who will often have had less experience of diabetes than the GPs they are presuming to advise. Diabetics value having a doctor involved in their care who is friendly and easy to talk to, and 85% of diabetics express a *preference* for management within general practice.[7]

A number of surveys have shown that organised care from general practice is every bit as effective as the care delivered from specialist hospital clinics,[7,38] so long as the GP care is properly structured.[39] These surveys have used surrogate measures of care such as glycaemic control and the adherence to clinical protocols rather than actual outcome measures, but now at least one survey from general practice has shown a reduced rate of admission to hospital among diabetics undergoing structured care.[40] It does not seem to matter much what form the structured care takes. The use of a protocol within the normal consultation framework,[39] the use of mini clinics (that is, designated separate clinics to care for diabetics)[38] and the 'Diabetic Day' where on one day a month a group of diabetics are invited to attend[41] seem equally effective ways of delivering care.

Diabetics suitable for complete care in general practice are:

- Those who are treated by diet alone
- Those who are treated by diet and tablets.

Diabetics requiring referral and/or shared care with the hospital are:

- Insulin-treated diabetics. Some practitioners may be happy to take on the full care of the well-controlled Type 1 diabetics
- Children
- Pregnant women and women planning to conceive
- Patients with known complications such as retinopathy, nephropathy and neuropathy.

Setting up structured diabetic care

Time and resources

A routine review attendance will take about 20 minutes if performed properly, and an annual check will take about 30 minutes if done all at once (in some mini clinics the diabetic is reviewed by a nurse, and then seen later by the doctor). If not enough time is allowed, the staff and patients will become frustrated, and a less-than-perfect job is done. Most of the tasks of diabetic care can be undertaken by appropriately trained *nursing colleagues*. Prescribing, fundoscopy and the more detailed neurological assessment is best done by a doctor. In some areas the fundoscopy is delegated to the local ophthalmic opticians to good effect. This level of involvement is clearly more than an average list patient would receive. It has been estimated that this extra care has a cost to general practice of around £4000 per GP per year (2000 prices).[42]

Develop a protocol

A written protocol for the practice and in particular for the diabetic care team has a number of advantages

- It consolidates team attitudes to diabetes
- It requires a literature search
- It provides a checklist for use in routine care
- It identifies training needs.

Practices which can show they are implementing an accepted protocol of care to their diabetics can claim sessional payments for the work.

Hunt the diabetic

In the absence of structured care up to a quarter of known diabetics do not get any diabetic follow-up.[7] Add to this the third of diabetics who are not yet diagnosed, and the importance of identification becomes clear. At first the known diabetics can be located from the practitioners' memory, and a review of the repeat prescribing records and disease index (if available). The list is then added to as patients present for review. New diabetics can be identified in the first instance by urinalysis:

- Opportunistically
- When risk factors are present
- New patient medicals
- Other medicals, for instance for insurance purposes

- Antenatal clinics
- Well person clinics.

Once identified, a diabetic can be offered an appointment in the appropriate clinic or surgery. Defaulters can be followed up with fresh appointments. The housebound can be visited.

Monitor progress

The performance of the care can be audited. Average blood sugar or HbA1c levels can be collated. Defaulters and lost patients can be reviewed. Hospital admissions can be monitored.

Summary

- One in fifty of the UK population have diabetes, two thirds of whom have been diagnosed
- Type 2 diabetes is more likely in the elderly and the obese. It is about 10 times commoner than Type 1 diabetes
- The risks of diabetes are due to the effect of the disease on both large and small blood vessels. Microvascular complications involve the eyes, kidneys and nerves
- The majority of diabetics die from cardiovascular disease
- Good control of blood pressure reduces the cardiovascular risk in diabetics. A target of 140/80 is advised
- Good glycaemic control reduces microvascular risks. A target HbA1c below 7% is advised
- All diabetics should be on a suitable diet. Diet alone is rarely sufficient to control the blood sugars, and most diabetics cheat on their diet
- Metformin reduces insulin resistance and are the first choice for overweight Type 2 diabetics. Dose is limited by gastrointestinal side effects
- Diabetics prefer to be followed up in primary care. Structured care can deliver results just as good as specialised hospital clinics
- Educating patients about their diabetes improves glycaemic control
- Good primary care diabetes management depends on teamwork

Topics for discussion

- It is more important to control a diabetic's blood pressure than blood sugar
- Now that the overlap in the care of hypertension, diabetes and coronary heart disease is so great, it makes sense in primary care to have a single clinic for all three diseases
- GPs are quite able to start insulin treatment
- The extra fee that GPs can claim for managing diabetes should be scrapped.

References

1. O'Rahilly S. Non-insulin dependent diabetes mellitus: the gathering storm. *BMJ* 1997; 314: 955–9.
2. Fry J. Diabetes. *Update* 1993; 46: 695–9.
3. Savage D. Diabetic emergencies in children. *Update* 1992; 45: 487–96.
4. Gardner S G, Bingley P J, Sawtell P A et al. Rising incidence of insulin dependent diabetes in children aged under 5 years in the Oxford region: time trend analysis. *BMJ* 1997; 315: 713–7.

5. Amiel S A. Non-insulin-dependent diabetes mellitus. *Update* 1994; 48: 256–65.
6. Liebson C, O'Brien P, Atkinson E et al. Relative contributions of incidence and survival to increasing prevalence of adult-onset diabetes mellitus: a population-based study. *Am J Epidemiol* 1997; 146: 12–22.
7. Balme M. Diabetes in general practice. Royal College of General Practitioners Members' Reference Book 1990, London; Sabrecrown: 1990.
8. Dobson R. Number of UK diabetic patients set to double by 2010. *BMJ* 2000; 320: 1029.
9. Donnelly R, Emslie-Smith A M, Gardner I D and Morris A D. *ABC of arterial and venous disease.* Vascular complications of diabetes. *BMJ* 2000; 320: 1062–66.
10. Mills K B. Diabetic retinopathy. Romford; Smith and Nephew Pharmaceuticals Ltd.
11. Flanagan D. Screening for diabetic retinopathy. *The Practitioner* 1994; 238: 37–42.
12. Ryder R. Screening for diabetic retinopathy. *BMJ* 1995; 311: 207–8.
13. Amiel S A. Insulin-dependant diabetes mellitus. *Update* 1994; 48: 421–7.
14. Kenny C J, Koperski M, Page M et al. GP Pocket Guide to NIDDM. London; Medical Imprint: 1995.
15. Minerva. *BMJ* 1997; 314: 1634.
16. Close C. Take action against diabetes. *Medical Monitor* 1997; 10(20): 54–6.
17. Minerva. *BMJ* 2001; 322: 564.
18. Minerva. *BMJ* 1996; 312: 1156.
19. The Expert Committee on the Diagnosis and Classification of Diabetes Mellitus. Report of the Expert Committee on the Diagnosis and Classification of Diabetes Mellitus. *Diabetes Care* 1997; 20: 1183–97.
20. The Diabetes Control and Complications Trial Research Group. The effects of intensive treatment of diabetes on the development and progression of long-term complications in insulin-dependent diabetes mellitus. *New Eng J Med* 1993; 329: 977–86.
21. UK Prospective Diabetes Study Group. Intensive blood-glucose control with sulphonylureas or insulin compared with conventional treatment and risk of complications in patients with Type 2 diabetes (UKPDS 33). *The Lancet* 1998; 352: 837–53.
22. Hermann W H on behalf of *Clinical Evidence.* Glycaemic control in diabetes. *BMJ* 1999; 319: 104–6.
23. Amiel S A. Diabetic control and complications. *BMJ* 1993; 307: 881–2.
24. British Diabetic Association. UKPDS. Implications for the care of people with Type 2 diabetes. London: BDA,1998.
25. Reducing long-term complications of Type 2 diabetes. *Drug and Therapeutics Bulletin* 1999; 37(11): 84–7.
26. Tuomilehto J. Controlling glucose and blood pressure in Type 2 diabetes. *BMJ* 2000; 321: 394–5.
27. British Cardiac Society, British Hyperlipidaemia Association, British Hypertension Society, British Diabetic Association. Joint British recommendations on prevention of coronary heart disease in clinical practice: summary. *BMJ* 2000; 320: 705–8.
28. Heller S, Connor H, Livingstone D et al. Type II Diabetes. *General Practitioner*, 27 November 1992.
29. Waine C, Tasker P, Gedney J et al. Royal College of General Practitioners: Guidelines for the care of patients with diabetes. London; RCGP: 1993.
30. Tate P. The Doctor's Communication Handbook. Abingdon: Radcliffe Medical Press, 1994.
31. Non-insulin-dependent diabetes mellitus (part 2). *MeReC Bulletin* 1996; 7: 29–32.

32. Singh D. Obesity in NIDDM. *Geriatric Medicine* 1996; 26(6): 42–5.
33. Non-insulin-dependent diabetes mellitus (part 1). *MeReC Bulletin* 1996; 7: 21–4.
34. National Institute for Clinical Excellence. Summary of Guidance Issued to the NHS in England and Wales. Volume 2 April 2001. London; DoH, 2001.
35. Davies T M E, Strong J A and Bloom S R. Compliance in diabetes mellitus: a self assessment study. *Practical Diabetes* 1988; 5(4): 170–2.
36. Evans J M M, Newton R W, Ruta D A et al. Frequency of blood glucose monitoring in relation to glycaemic control: observational study with diabetes database. *BMJ* 1999; 319: 83–6.
37. What diabetic care to expect. London; British Diabetic Association: 1989.
38. Parnell S J, Zalin A M and Clarke C W F. Care of diabetic patients in hospital clinics and general practice clinics: a study in Dudley. *Br J Gen Pract* 1993; 43: 65–9.
39. Foulkes A, Kinmouth A, Frost S et al. Organised personal care an effective choice for managing diabetes in general practice. *J Roy Coll Gen Pract* 1989; 39: 444–7.
40. Farmer A and Coulter A. Organisation of care for diabetic patients in general practice: influence on hospital admissions. *Br J Gen Pract* 1990; 40: 56–8.
41. Koperski M. How effective is systematic care of diabetic patients? A study in one general practice. *Br J Gen Pract* 1992; 42: 508–11.
42. Anon. GPs need £4000 each to offer the best service. *General Practitioner* April 28 2000: 12.

Exercise

Tutorial aims	The registrar is able to:
	• **Identify list patients who will benefit from increasing their physical activity**
	• **Make personalised recommendations for an exercise programme.**
Learning objectives	By the end of the tutorial the registrar can:
	• List five benefits of exercise in primary prevention
	• List five benefits of exercise in secondary prevention
	• List three benefits of exercise in tertiary prevention
	• Describe an exercise programme for a patient with angina
	• Describe an exercise programme for a patient with osteoporosis
	• Discuss the GP's role in exercise promotion.

Introduction

The notion that physical exercise is good for people is relatively new. Traditionally hard physical work has been associated with being poor and of low social status: rich people get poor people to do their work for them. The majority of jobs involved physical labour until the Industrial Revolution and the rise of the machine, since there was little alternative. Devices are 'labour-saving'. When people get rich they retire from work. The whole thrust of industrial development has been to prevent the toils of the past. Now the backlash has arrived. Lack of sufficient exercise is a risk factor for all sorts of human ills. For example, the prevalence of risk factors for coronary heart disease is[1]

Cigarette smoking	30%
Hypertension	15%
Hyperlipidaemia	30%
Lack of physical exercise	70%

The level of risk from each of these factors is approximately equivalent.[2]

Is there a problem?

Children score best on measures of fitness, but few experience regular levels of physical activity sufficient to stress their heart and lungs appropriately. In

England and Wales there has been a decline in physical activity among two-to seven-year-olds: 33% of boys and 38% of girls are not reaching recommended activity guidelines.[3] Just under half of children under age 16 spend more than two hours a week in physical education lessons, but even this is twice as much as the 17- and 18-year-olds. Boys are more energetic than girls.[4] The government has responded with a report: *Raising the game*. This proposes a minimum of two hours' physical education a week for children under age 16, with an emphasis on competitive sports and team games. The emphasis on competition is unfortunate: many schoolchildren are put off sport for ever because they are not good enough to make the team. Childhood exercise levels predict those in later life.[4] *Adults* in general get less exercise than children.

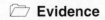 **Evidence**

The Allied Dunbar national fitness survey[5]		
Men and women aged 16 to 74, most of whom regarded themselves as physically fit		
	Men (%)	Women (%)
Insufficient exercise for cardiovascular benefit	70	80
Unable to sustain a walk up a 5% gradient at 3 mph	35	65
Many people over age 55 have insufficient strength to perform some tasks of daily living.		

The *elderly* have potentially the most to gain from improving their fitness. They are more likely to have the illnesses which are ameliorated by exercise, and are more likely to benefit from improved mobility and stamina.

Evidence

Fitness in the elderly[6]
In the over-60 age group:
• 90% are unable to walk on level ground at 2.5 mph (the speed required to cross a pelican crossing in time)
• 60% of women do not have sufficient strength in their legs to get up from a chair without using their hands.

A study from Norfolk of people aged 45 to 74 found that a tenth engage in no physical recreational activity at all, a third never climb any stairs in their normal lives, and that the median time spent watching television is about 22 hours a week with a tenth of people watching for over 30 hours a week.[7]

The benefits of exercise

Physical exercise is promoted for the primary and secondary prevention of a wide range of physical[1] and psychological illness.[8] The benefits of fitness are seen in both sexes and at all ages. Improved fitness can also be of benefit in the tertiary prevention of disability. Even the effects of ageing itself can be slowed by regular exercise.[9] There is still some controversy about the *quality of the evidence* supporting the benefits of exercise.[10] Most studies have been retrospective, and so it may be that healthy people also like to exercise. Longitudinal cohort studies have confirmed the benefit of becoming fit having been unfit,[11] but there remains the concern that the unhealthy may be less likely to be retained in a fitness programme.

Vascular benefits

Sedentary lifestyle is the most prevalent alterable risk factor for cardiovascular disease.[1] The *British Regional Heart Survey* on men aged 40 to 59 found that moderate levels of activity gave primary protection against *stroke* (50% reduction) and *heart attack* (60% reduction). More vigorous exercise did not seem to confer increased benefit, and was actually found to be quite dangerous in those with a history of stroke or heart attack. A survey of men and women of all ages found that the least fit men had eight times the death rate for cardiovascular disease compared to the most fit. The trend in women was less pronounced.[12]

Exercise training *after a heart attack* reduces the risk of further heart attack and death from heart failure by 25%.[13] This is proportionately a considerable benefit, as the risk of a heart attack in a patient who has already had one is much higher than in a patient who does not have known coronary heart disease. Regular physical activity reduces both systolic and diastolic *blood pressure*. The active can expect a reduction of 10/8 mmHg,[14] a significant benefit but not enough to make other treatments redundant.

It is quite plausible that regular exercise should provide primary and secondary protection against cardiovascular events. Regular exercise increases the *high density lipoprotein* level and reduces the triglyceride level.[15] Weight may also be controlled, and stopping smoking may be easier. Blood pressure is reduced. There may also be effects on blood, making it less likely to clot.[13] As the person gets fitter, they are able to exercise for longer. After a cardiovascular event, exercise reduces blood pressure and improves muscle perfusion so reducing vascular resistance. The overall effect is to reduce cardiac work. In addition the *electrical stability* of the heart is improved, and there is less response to adrenaline, making arrhythmia less likely.[14]

Osteoporosis

Physical activity *up to the age of 20* is directly related to maximum bone mass, and hence the risk of osteoporotic fracture.[16] Women of all ages between 20 and 80 who exercise at least *three times a week* have a higher bone density than those who are sedentary.[17] Exercise reduces the risk of hip fracture by about half, but it has to be *weight bearing* exercise: swimming is less effective.[18] Osteoporotic fractures occur because people fall over. Improved flexibility, balance and the nimbleness to correct the occasional stumble all reduce the risk of falls. Ironically, fit people are more likely to put themselves into situations where falls occur: sitting in an armchair is less immediately hazardous than abseiling down an Alp.

Other physical illness

• Exercise improves *glucose tolerance and increases insulin sensitivity.*[14]

The prevalence of non-insulin-dependent diabetes is accordingly reduced in the physically active. There are also benefits in weight control.

- Physical activity protects against colonic *cancer* and probably against breast cancer. Exercise does not seem to make any type of cancer more common.[19]
- In the chronically disabled, a group which includes many of the elderly, regular exercise reduces the *level of handicap*. In rheumatic complaints exercise may reduce the pain and swelling in the joints.[9]
- Exercise improves balance and flexibility, and so reduces the *risk of falls.*[16] The National Service Framework for Elderly People has highlighted the problem of falls for special attention.
- Exercise reduces *disability* in

  intermittent claudication
  heart failure
  angina
  asthma
  chronic obstructive pulmonary disease

- Improved *mobility* reduces the risk of

  faecal impaction
  incontinence
  deep vein thrombosis
  pulmonary embolism
  gravitational oedema
  skin ulceration

Improving ability to get out of the house reduces *loneliness*.

Mental illness

- In mild to moderate *depression*, regular exercise is at least as helpful as cognitive therapy and behavioural therapy. In major depression, exercise reduces symptoms significantly, and has a quicker effect than other treatments. Exercise provides primary protection against depression in women but not in men. Exercise does, however, reduce relapse rates in depressed men: this sex difference is unexplained.[8]
- *Anxiety* is helped by regular exercise. The exercise should be aerobic, non-competitive, predictable and rhythmic.[8]
- Increased exercise helps to internalise the *locus of control.*[20]

How much exercise?

🖹 Guidelines

Exercise for general health promotion[21]

Recommendation of the Health Education Authority

- Five 30-minute or ten 15-minute periods of exercise a week
- Suitable exercises are

  brisk walking

gardening
cycling
swimming

This recommendation is a *compromise*, because

- The evidence for the prevention of *cardiovascular* events suggests that in a week three 30-minute periods of moderately intense physical activity are best. The vigour of the exercise should be enough to achieve a pulse rate of 50% above normal.[13] In the previously sedentary this can usually be achieved by walking at a pace of one mile every 15 minutes.[15] As fitness increases, the pace can also increase.
- Preventing *osteoporosis* requires weight-bearing exercise, so that swimming and cycling are less useful. High impact exercises include jogging, step aerobics and football, but benefit may also be apparent from lower impact exercise such as dancing, gardening or golf.[7]
- *Weight control* requires the expenditure of energy over several hours, such as a game of golf, but this is not much use for cardiovascular protection.

While the goals for healthy exercise levels remain a little confused, it can be asserted with some confidence that *nearly all people*, of whatever age or level of disability (with a very few exceptions), *will get a health benefit from increasing their exercise levels*. To a large extent the benefits are linearly related to the amount of exercise done: even a bit of exercise is better than no exercise at all, and a lot of exercise is (up to a point) better than a little exercise.[16]

Fit to drop?

Some early and well-publicised reports suggested that vigorous exercise leads to sudden coronary death.

- The overall chance of cardiac arrest in active men is only 40% of that in sedentary men[15]
- During exercise the risk of death increases up to sixfold, but the risk while not exercising (the majority of the time) is halved[16]
- Sudden vigorous and unaccustomed exercise is potentially hazardous for middle-aged and older people,[15] but moderate and even vigorous exercise is still a good idea when the person is trained up gradually for it.

▤ Guidelines

When not to exercise:[2]

- During an infection which causes fever or myalgia
- During extreme climatic conditions
- When very breathless or distressed
- Just after a large meal.

To prevent injury, people should *warm up* before exercise and *warm down* after. Tissues such as muscle, tendon, ligament and bone adapt to exercise more slowly than the cardiorespiratory system.[22] A few minutes bending and stretching beforehand and a few minutes stretching and walking afterwards are all that is needed. Regular moderate exercise causes less injury and does just as much good as the brief and frantic variety. Some people, especially the elderly, will contact their GP to see if they are *medically fit* to begin exercising. For them, checking the blood pressure and asking specifically about ischaemic chest pain is all that is required. There are very few chronic conditions, with the possible exception of unstable angina, in which exercise is not a good idea. Nevertheless the duration and pace of the chosen exercise should be built up to gradually over weeks and months.

📄 **Guidelines**   **The modified fitness activity readiness questionnaire (PAR-Q test)[22]**

- Are you over age 60?
- Do you get chest pains?
- Do you get breathlessness or dizziness?
- Do you have diabetes?
- Do you have a heart condition/heart murmur/had heart surgery?
- Have you been told you have high blood pressure?
- Do you smoke?
- Do you suffer from blackouts?

- If chest pain, palpitation, severe breathlessness, fainting or blurred vision occur during the exercise, then the patient should stop and go back to the GP for a little chat
- Some types of exercise are unsuitable for some people. For instance arthritis may be worsened by impact during jogging: swimming is a better bet. Patients with angina should not be out shovelling snow in the cold
- Patients with controlled epilepsy and asthma can get involved in regulated exercise
- Patients with back pain benefit from exercise, but they are best advised to avoid impact exercises and try swimming.

Checking whether a diabetic is fit to exercise is a little more complicated because of the cluster of other cardiovascular risks which diabetics tend to have as well as their diabetes: obesity, hypertension, previous vascular events etc. For patients over age 35 or who have had diabetes a long time an ECG or an exercise ECG should be done to look for ischaemia. Blood sugar should be tested before and after exercise. Accessible carbohydrate should be carried during exercise.[16]

📄 **Guidelines**   **Fitness after injury[23]**

- Are you able to move the injured part fully without pain or stiffness?
- Does stretching the surrounding muscles cause pain?
- Are coordination and balance back to normal?

- Is resisted movement painful?
- Is there pain, stiffness or swelling after exercise?
- Are you confident the injury has healed?
- Do you know what caused the injury, and will it happen again?

Why don't people exercise more?

The *drop-out* rate from exercise programmes is high at 50%. Cognitive and behavioural strategies may help another 20% stay the course: suitable, explicit and challenging *goals can be agreed* such as attending aerobics three times a week or jogging round the grounds twice in 30 minutes. Setting unrealistic goals worsens the risk of dropout.[16] Generally time goals are better than distance goals for achieving improvement.[8]

The main reason why, people say, they do not exercise is lack of time.[5] Other reasons may include

- *Childhood experience.* Active children carry their exercise habits into adult life[4]
- *Facilities.* School sports facilities are not as good as they might be. Some schools have been forced to sell off playing fields for financial reasons. This reduces the access of children to exercise. For the adult, exercise costs *money*. There are entry fees to swimming baths and gymnasia, and then there is the necessary equipment. Cycling is excellent exercise, but you need a bicycle and somewhere safe to ride it
- *Culture of participation.* Exercise is a minority activity. It is not usual to play sport or exercise as an adult. The government and the media clearly have a role to play here
- *Gymnasium culture.* Leisure clubs are assumed to be full of overdeveloped body-builders who are obsessional about their exercise regimes. They may be in the minority, but they are always at the gym and so seem to be a permanent feature. The *clothing* normally worn is not particularly flattering for the overweight, and there are always a few perfect body specimens for depressing comparison. The use of anabolic steroids is widespread: 6% of men and 1.4% of women who attend gyms, and up to 60% of attenders at needle exchanges, are users[24]
- *Culture of excellence.* Top-flight athletes are not physiologically normal. Much of their ability is the result of training, but much is a result of heredity. Most people are not physiologically capable of running a mile in under four minutes. The emphasis of the media on sporting excellence portrays images that few can emulate. This can put off those who will 'never be any good' at sport: these are often the people in most urgent need of more exercise.

Helping patients to exercise more

The Allied Dunbar survey found that a majority of adults understood the benefits of exercise and thought they were physically fit when in fact they were not. Only half of the sedentary elderly (over 65) have any intention of trying to increase their levels of exercise.[21] The general practitioner has a number of options.

Option: do nothing

Most of the factors which determine how much people exercise are outside the control of doctors. They are to do with the availability of facilities, how sport is marketed and public attitudes to leisure. These are responsibilities for governments, not doctors. On the other hand, pro-active health promotion is increasingly seen as the proper concern of the health service, and much worthwhile prevention can potentially be achieved by the encouragement of exercise.

Option: set a good example

Whether they feel comfortable about it or not, doctors still have a measure of social status which should be used and not abused. Just as it is not good professionalism to be carried home drunk from the pub every night, GPs can by their own example encourage a more healthy lifestyle among their patients. You could attend the local swimming baths, or be seen cycling or jogging round the practice area. If other local agencies are holding events which encourage healthier lifestyles, a visit from and participation by the local GP can only help. Some practices have been known to organise their own fun run or sports day.

Option: prescribe exercise

The last few years have seen a number of schemes arranged whereby patients can get cheap access to local recreational facilities if recommended by their GP. In some cases the leisure centres involved cooperate in order to get the extra customers, and publicly to demonstrate their commitment to a higher calling than just profit. In other instances there may be subsidies from the health authority or social services department. Analysis of the existing schemes suggests that there are benefits, but modest ones. The efficacy of the schemes is roughly comparable to that of weight reduction and smoking cessation programmes; but their community effect is likely to be greater because primarily sedentary people outnumber smokers or the obese. Participants tend to *benefit more psychosocially than physically* from their involvement.[25]

Option: opportunistic exercise promotion

Parts of some elements of GP funding currently rely on the assessment of physical activity levels, for instance the New Patient Medical. Gathering the data is a good start, but is less useful if it is not accompanied by efforts to alter unhealthy habits. When diagnoses such as heart disease or diabetes are made, it is sensible to include exercise in the package of appropriate lifestyle recommendations.

Option: exercise clinic

Many health promotion clinics in general practice already routinely include the promotion of exercise. The exercise clinic is directed more specifically at increasing physical activity, and can also be available for patients who want to become more fit for general health reasons and not because they are already ill. The provisions of the clinic might be:

- Assessment of fitness to exercise
- Recommending personalised exercise programmes
- Follow-up of progress on the programme
- Sports injury service.

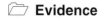 **Evidence**

> **Energy equivalents[22]**
>
> One hundred kilocalories of energy are used in:
>
> - 10 minutes running or cycling
> - 12 minutes swimming
> - 15 minutes squash or tennis
> - 30 minutes slow walking
> - 18 minutes fast walking
> - 20 to 25 minutes gardening
> - 75 minutes of fidgeting.[26]

Summary

- A third of children and four fifths of adults in the United Kingdom do not get enough exercise
- Insufficient exercise is as much a risk factor for cardiovascular disease as hypertension, smoking and raised cholesterol, but is more than twice as prevalent as any one of them
- The data confirming the benefits of exercise are not beyond criticism. It is possible, for instance, that healthy people like to exercise more than unhealthy ones
- Increasing exercise is of benefit in vascular disease, osteoporosis, diabetes, rheumatic complaints, depression and anxiety. Exercise also protects against immobility and some cancers
- The amount and type of exercise which is beneficial depends on the aims of the exercise. Cardiovascular fitness is improved by regular episodes of exercise designed to increase the heart rate. Osteoporosis prevention is best achieved by impact exercise. As a general principle, any exercise is better than no exercise, and more exercise is better than less
- Increasing exercise is safe for nearly everybody as long as there are no symptoms of existing cardiovascular disease. Diabetics, however, need special care
- Most of the reasons why people do not exercise more are not subject to medical control
- Half of sedentary people say they want to increase their exercise levels, and a GP can take a number of steps to encourage them. However, attempts to encourage people to increase their levels of exercise are frequently not successful.

Topics for discussion

- Suggest ways of dealing with the patient comment 'I can't exercise because I am too fat'
- Suggest ways of dealing with the patient comment; 'I needn't exercise because I am not overweight'
- The government should put at least as much resource into getting people to exercise more as it does into getting them to stop smoking
- Encouraging exercise is an underused treatment for anxiety and depression
- Your Primary Care Trust is offering the practice funds to encourage exercise.

How would you spend the money?

Which patients would you target?

• What would a practice policy on exercise contain?

📖 References

1. Smith F and Iliffe S. Exercise prescription in primary care. *Br J Gen Pract* 1997; 47: 272–3.
2. Todd D B. Prescription of exercise. *Update* 1996; 52: 408–11.
3. UK children take too little exercise. In Brief *BMJ* 2000; 320: 1558.
4. Trippe H. Children and sport. *BMJ* 1996; 312: 199–200.
5. Activity and Health Research. Allied Dunbar national fitness survey. London: Health Education Council and Sports Council, 1992.
6. Bird W. How 'healthy walks' have improved patients' fitness. *General Practitioner*, November 27 1998: 71–2.
7. Jakes R W, Khaw K-T, Day N E *et al.* Patterns of physical activity and ultrasound attenuation by heel bone among Norfolk cohort of European Prospective Investigation of Cancer (EPIC Norfolk): population based study. *BMJ* 2001; 322: 140–3.
8. Smeaton J. Physical exercise and mental health. *Psychiatry in Practice* 1995; 14(3): 16–18.
9. Young A and Dinan S. Fitness for older people. *BMJ* 1994; 309: 331–4.
10. MacAuley D. Exercise and health promotion. *Br J Gen Pract* 1993; 43: 443–4.
11. Blair S N, Kohl H W 3rd, Barlow C E et al. Changes in physical fitness and all-cause mortality. A prospective study of healthy and unhealthy men. *JAMA* 1995; 273: 1093–8.
12. Brodie D. GPs should promote the benefits of exercise. *Monitor Weekly,* 15 September 1993: 41–2.
13. Dargie H J and Grant S. Exercise. *BMJ* 1991; 303: 910–12.
14. Fentem P H. Benefits of exercise in health and disease. *BMJ* 1994; 308: 1291–5.
15. Hardman A. Exercise and the heart: Report of the British Heart Foundation Working Group. London: BHF, 1993.
16. Higgins R. 'Doctor, am I fit enough to exercise?' *The Practitioner* 2000; 244: 574–79.
17. Talmage R V, Stinnett S S, Landwehr J T et al. Age-related loss of mineral bone density in non-athletic and athletic women. *Bone Miner* 1986; 1: 115–25.
18. Law M R, Wald N J and Meade T W. Strategies for prevention of osteoporosis and hip fracture. *BMJ* 1991; 303: 453–9.
19. Batty D and Thune I. Does physical activity prevent cancer? *BMJ* 2000; 321: 1424–5.
20. See Tai S, Gould M and Iliffe S. Promoting healthy exercise among older people in general practice: issues in designing and evaluating therapeutic interventions. *Br J Gen Pract* 1997; 47: 119–22.
21. Powell K E and Pratt M. Physical activity and health. *BMJ* 1996; 313: 126–7.
22. Budgett R. Physical fitness. *General Practitioner* October 21 1994: 37–44.
23. Carroll S. Exercise: when is it safe for patients? *Modern Medicine* 1989; 34: 397–400.
24. Dawson R T. Drugs in sport: a new approach. *The Practitioner* 2000; 244: 1003.
25. Riddoch C. How effective are exercise schemes? *Update* 1999; 58: 1049.
26. Minerva *BMJ* 2000; 321: 1540.

Getting a job as a general practitioner principal

Tutorial aim	**The registrar is able to apply for a job as a general practice principal.**
Learning objectives	By the end of the tutorial the registrar can: • Find and select a suitable job vacancy • Write an appropriate CV • Write a covering letter • List required information about a practice • Describe an approach to being interviewed • List common pitfalls on entering a practice • Find out from practice accounts what the job will earn.

Background

General practice undergoes cycles of popularity as far as new medical graduates are concerned. Each reorganisation has the GP establishment complaining that things will never be the same again, and such protests resonate through the medical schools to deter prospective GPs. Ironically, the reduced recruitment provoked by the laments of the profession tends to worsen the situation.

> *The good news is that, whatever administrative hoops general practitioners are being asked to jump through, the job remains much the same. Patients are as delightful, demanding and exasperating as ever, general practitioners remain resourceful and dedicated professionals, and primary care teams have found the capacity to manage the ever more complex administrative and computer systems sent to try them[1]*

General practice is by some margin the biggest specialty within medicine. In 1997 there were 27 100 unrestricted principals in England.[2] The average list size per GP continues to fall – 1846 per full-time principal in England in 2001.[3] However, the British Medical Association points to trends which imply that a GP personpower crisis is just around the corner:

• Only 26% of United Kingdom medical graduates in 1993 *wanted* to enter general practice,[4] whereas over half of all graduates are needed. This may not be as bad as it sounds: four years on only 60% of male and under 50% of female doctors are in the specialty they chose at registration[4]

- The Joint Committee on Postgraduate Training for General Practice (JCPTGP) issued 1689 *certificates* in 2000,[5] a little better than the nadir of 1636 in 1998 which was the lowest number since 1981.[6] However, only 1229 GPs entered or re-entered general practice in 1999, the lowest for 10 years[7]
- There is a trend towards *earlier retirement* among GPs: only just over 1000 GPs are over age 60.[8] Three quarters of recently qualified GPs intend to retire before the age of 60, and a quarter expect to retire between ages 50 and 55[9]
- GPs are increasingly opting for *less than full-time* practice: a third of GPs are non-principals, nearly two thirds of whom work under 25 hours a week.[9] Women now comprise 34% of all GPs.[7] Official figures may not reflect the real situation: a GP has only to contract for 26 hours a week to be considered 'full-time' and so claim full practice allowances
- Many of the *Commonwealth graduates* recruited in the 1960s into general practice are now reaching retirement age and because of European Union regulations cannot be replaced from that source.[10]

The doctor who wants to enter general practice should have plenty of choice. There is a GP shortage of up to 12% in some areas of the country.[10] However, each GP vacancy attracts 8.5 applicants, and 89% are filled within six months.[1]

What do registrars want?

 Evidence

Intentions of GP registrars[11]

A survey of 140 delegates at the seventh National GP Trainee Conference in June 1993:

Straight into work as a GP principal	24%
Locum work	30%
More hospital work	11%
Work abroad	30%
Leave medicine temporarily	11%
Leave medicine permanently	1.5%
Join associated medical field	3.5%

This will be of particular concern to government as each GP costs about £180000 to train[12] (1994 prices = £240840 in 2001).

Around half of registrars say they are looking for a job in a suburban area and 40% in a rural location: only 8.5% are looking for a practice in the inner city. Thirty five per cent of registrars are looking for job-sharing posts.[11] A further survey of registrars in the North West Thames region found that 28% would consider working in inner London. Twelve per cent said they would be prepared for single-handed practice, and 28% would work in a practice of two.[13]

What is your ideal practice like?

The first and probably the most difficult part of finding a practice is to decide what sort of practice you are looking for. Many registrars have experience during their training of at most two practices, and since these are training practices which will have had to reach particular standards to qualify to train, they are not like other general practices. There is a tendency for registrars to want a practice like their training practice – the *clone effect*. A major advantage of doing locum work after vocational training is that not only do you see other practices from the inside, but you also buy time to look around the options. It is important to choose a practice *carefully*. A full-time GP will spend more time at work than with their spouse and this indicates the level of carefulness that is appropriate. No practice will fit exactly to your requirements, but there will be some things you are prepared to compromise on (desired factors) and some things on which you will not (mandatory factors). Factors to be taken into account when choosing a practice are:[14]

- *Practice area*. The work and the social role of a GP can be very different working in a rural area from urban practice. Rural practice means having to display a wider range of clinical skills as there is less ready back-up from hospitals and the ambulance services. There will probably be more travelling which may make the workload very heavy from time to time. A practice with a base in an agreeable area may have patients in the less salubrious parts of town or country, or may have little pockets within the area where problems tend to be focused
- *Partner number*. Small partnerships can be more friendly, and there is usually less inertia when practice changes are needed. There is usually more continuity of patient care. On the other hand interpersonal squabbles become magnified. With fewer partners there are greater workload fluctuations when a partner is absent
- *Patient number*. Dividing the total list size by the number of doctors gives a bare idea of workload. A sight of a map of the practice boundaries will show how dispersed the patients are, giving an indication of problems with home visits. It is a good idea to look at the appointment book and the home and emergency visit logs
- *Partner characteristics*. The age range, sex and special interests of the other partners will give an idea of what the practice is short of in terms of GP skills. The age structure will show whether any more partners are due to leave. An old-style autocratic senior-partner-run practice may (but not always) be intolerant of change and development. If all the partners have lots of outside interests and are pursuing 'portfolio careers', then their availability to do the practice work is less. Academic partners invariably have better things to do than see patients
- *Premises*. Practice-owned buildings have to be bought into, so money has to be found. If the practice dispenses this will add an average of £80 000 to the buying-in costs[15] (1994 prices = £107 040 in 2001). Working from more than one site provides additional challenges
- *Income*. The list size and the achievement of targets will give a broad indication of likely income. Income will also depend on starting share, time to parity and the buying-in arrangements. The time to insist on seeing the books is not, however, until after the interviews

- *Workload*. The way the on-call is organised can make a difference to workload and income. Deputising services and cooperatives can ease the workload burden considerably, but are expensive. Inequitable work sharing causes problems and resentment. There may be differences between partners in the number of surgeries or amount of on-call being done, often justified only by tradition. Is there a shared list or are there personal lists?
- *Organisation*. The practice manager is invariably pivotal in the way the practice works, and the character of the manager is thus of importance. A practice deed should exist and be in good order. The practice deed will have to be changed to accommodate the new partner anyway, so this is a good time to update the deed generally. The existence of clinics and ancillary staff should be checked, as well as any problems with staff members. Does the overall practice philosophy accord with your own? How well does the practice work within their Primary Care Group/Trust?
- *Local hospitals*. The availability of a range of secondary care facilities and investigative procedures can make a big difference to the pattern of work. The presence of adequate postgraduate education facilities is desirable
- *Local amenities*. Will you and your family enjoy living in or around the practice area? What are the schools, cultural and leisure facilities like?
- *Vacancy*. How has the vacancy arisen? Has a partner left, and if so why? Are there internal partnership tensions?

You will get a rough insight into these areas through looking round and informal discussions. The time to get into more detail is at interview.

Finding a job vacancy

It is usually easier to find out about job vacancies which arise in the area you are already working in. You will have contacts and will have established a reputation. You will also be seen to be committed to the area and so less likely to want to move on. A third of registrars get a job without making an application at all.[16] Sources of information are:

- Adverts in the British Medical Journal, British Journal of General Practice or one of the free medical newspapers
- Word of mouth from colleagues or course organisers
- The Health Authority will know of posts falling vacant, especially single-handed posts. Some will offer to circulate your CV for you
- The Local Medical Committee (LMC) will often be prepared to help
- Advertisements in the local Postgraduate Centre.

Getting short-listed

It helps if you already know the practice and they know you. Make sure that any other information they have about you works to your advantage. The important thing is to create a good impression.

Before the application, find out as much as you can about the practice and the area. This helps you make a choice, and also informs your application. Talking to people in the local pubs and shops can be illuminating.

Contact the practice and ask to visit. If you have visited, ring up later to thank them and express your continuing interest.

If a *locum* becomes available in a target practice, try to do it. You will get a much better idea of how the practice works, and it is also a good chance to get yourself known by the partners and, perhaps as important, by the rest of the practice staff.

The curriculum vitae

This may be the first information the practice will have about you. It will arrive along with a variable number of others, and time spent on presentation will make it stand out from the rest. Try to make it well spaced out and legibly printed. Access to a word processor is extremely useful as lots of good quality copies can be made, and it is also possible to alter the text for each application. Use lots of headings. Be concise.

Your work career so far should get the most attention and detail. Do not try to cover any gaps as they are very easy to spot. If you spent a few months being ill, or climbing in the Himalayas, then say so. It might even help – a consumer's view of the NHS can be quite instructive.

The front page of your CV is the most accessible and should include nearly all the relevant information, even if this is expanded later in the text. Suitable items for the front page are:[17]

- *Personal details:* Name in full, address, date of birth, marital status, spouse's career, children, nationality. Confirmation that you hold a driving licence. General Medical Council registration number. Defence society membership number
- *Education:* A chronological list[18] from A levels (including grades only if they are very good) to graduation, including any prizes
- *Work background:* This is traditionally listed backwards with the present job first.[15] Aspects of the jobs relevant to general practice, and especially any relevant to the target practice, can be highlighted. Irrelevant items will obscure the message. *Positive* and active words will stand out more: *achieved, improved, successful, developed* and *created* are better words than *did.* For most registrars the most relevant work experience will be related to their training practice. Include details of eligibility for the *lists*: obstetric, minor surgery, child health surveillance
- *Other interests:* Only list the ones you are particularly keen on
- *Referees:* It looks odd if you do not include your trainer as a referee.

In the ensuing text, topics can be expanded. Remember, however, that more than three pages of even the brightest prose is unlikely to be read fully.

If you must include a photograph, it should be an original print, and a reasonably accurate likeness. Photocopies of photographs and the little passport-sized items which you get from the machine in Woolworth's always make you look like the registrar from hell. Have due regard to the aesthetic sensitivities of your putative partners.

The covering letter

The covering letter is the main way of impressing the partners. It is traditionally written by hand, but this is now less important (unless the advert specifically requests it). Try to think what you would want to know if you wanted a new partner. Competence is often assumed from the training and any further qualifications, so this is only part of the issue.

Connections with the area go down well. If you know the area already, and have other reasons to stay, you are more likely to stick with the job. The commonest time for a partnership to break down is in the early years. Frequent changes in partnership take up a lot of time and are stressful. Your research of the area may have given you some extra insights into the *problems* and *possibilities* the practice may have. Include these in your letter. It might be worth making the odd suggestion about the future of the practice, but err on the side of caution as the other partners will always know more about the problems and possibilities than you do.

Tell them *why you want to go into general practice*, and why you want to join them. All GPs think their way is best, and have invested a lot of effort in getting things the way they are. Stroke a few egos.

Include something about *non-medical interests*. The zealot is regarded with suspicion, but then so is the laggard. Don't exaggerate: sooner or later you will come across a real expert who will easily call your bluff.

Show them you have at least read the advert. Try to *address any issues specifically raised* (e.g. 'eligible for obstetric list') and indicate how you would deal with them. Faced with a pile of nearly identical applications, most GPs will at first look for ways of reducing the number. Failure to comply with a condition in the advert is a good way of getting your application binned.

Working in a general practice involves much more than just seeing the patients. Any interests or *special experience* you may have in administrative or personnel areas should be covered in either the CV or the letter.

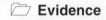 **Evidence**

What do partnerships look for?[19]

In a study in 1993, 110 GPs in the North West region were asked what qualities they would look for in a new partner[19]

- 75% preferred an applicant under 35 years old, and 57% preferred a married applicant. Children were thought an advantage by 45%
- 35% wanted an innovative partner, and 20% wanted an extrovert while only 8% wanted an introvert
- 65% expected some postgraduate qualifications, of which MRCGP and DRCOG were favourites. However 20% felt that too many qualifications would be a disadvantage
- 30% preferred a local applicant, and 55% would appoint their own registrar
- Postgraduate experience in obstetrics/gynaecology, paediatrics and general medicine was seen as desirable by over 80% of appointing GPs
- 65% of practices put adverts in the press six months or more before the vacancy arose, so the aspirant partner should plan early.

Behaviour at interview

Once short-listed you will be required to attend one or a number of interview situations. You are being assessed during them all, even during the trial by sherry. Be on time and look the part but *be yourself* as far as the circumstances will allow. Joining a practice is making a contract, not winning a prize. A successful recruitment process is one after which you can work with the partnership and they can work with you. If you create a false impression which you cannot or do not intend to sustain then they will get a distorted idea of you and you of them. This will inevitably lead to strains in the relationship.

The partnership will be looking for someone who will fit in with them. *Philosophical and religious views* are usually strongly held: if you or the practice have particularly strong beliefs in areas which may affect the day-to-day work of the practice, then it is as well to get them out into the open at an early stage. Disagreement on such things can lead to a lot of future problems, and it is no good hoping you can convert them all.

Listen to the questions, and try to answer them. Most GPs don't have the faintest idea how to interview, and may well be as nervous as you are. Those who are organised will have looked carefully at what they think the practice needs in a new partner, and will be looking for someone to fulfil those needs. It may be possible from your research to predict what characteristics are being looked for and to respond accordingly.

The best predictor of future behaviour is past behaviour. Interviewers with any sense will spend most of the time discussing your current job, finding out what qualities you have used and how you coped with problems. *Short anecdotes are more memorable* than bare information,[20] and also indicate that you can deliver what you say you can deliver. To a question such as 'How well do you cope with depression?', you could reply 'I think I cope reasonably well'. More memorably you could reply 'This is how I coped with a depressed patient I saw recently . . .', and go on to tell the story.

You are interviewing them as much as they are interviewing you. You will need to know certain things about the practice, and a checklist does not go amiss. Many of the questions may well have been answered in informal discussion, but you will need some information on all of the following.[21]

How do things work?

- How many GPs and staff are there?
- How is the workload shared out? Try to look at the appointment diary and the visits list
- What is the list size, and are any changes expected?
- How is out-of-hours cover organised? Cooperative, deputising, rota etc.
- What attached staff are there?
- Are the practice annual reports available?
- Who is in the practice's PCG/T?
- Are any specialist services offered?
- Scope for outside appointments?
- Does the practice dispense?
- Is the practice computerised and are there links with the health authority?

- Any special allowances e.g. deprivation?
- What sort of medical records are used? Can they be viewed?

Money

- How many years to parity?
- What are the profit-sharing arrangements?
- Any special clauses in agreement, e.g. building up own list?
- Are all earnings pooled: outside jobs, seniority, PGEA?
- Provision for maternity/paternity leave?
- Can you see the practice accounts?
- Who owns the premises?
- What are the buying-in arrangements? How are valuations made?

Philosophy

- How are relations with local providers?
- Is the health authority regarded as helpful or obstructive?
- Are higher targets being met, e.g. child health surveillance?
- Are team meetings held?
- Is it a training practice?
- What is the attitude toward staff training?
- Any plans for a nurse practitioner?
- Any prescribing policies? Practice formulary
- What is the attitude towards private patients?
- How are practice decisions made?
- What is the attitude towards external advice e.g. management consultants?
- What are the audit arrangements?
- Any provision for sabbaticals and study leave?
- Is the practice keen to innovate?

Lifestyle

- What are property costs like?
- What are local schools like?
- How many partners have children?
- Any sporting or leisure facilities available?

Should you be concerned about money?

Yes, you should. You are entering a business venture. Everyone else will be acutely concerned with making a living, and in a partnership you have responsibilities to your partners as well as to yourself.

Working out your earnings

When you have been offered a post, it is important to look at the practice accounts before accepting. They should be shown to your own accountant for an assessment. If the accounts are not forthcoming or are not for the latest available year, then either mismanagement or a deception may be assumed. There may be undisclosed debts which need to be serviced. The post is unacceptable.

Profit share and time to parity should be laid down in the partnership deed, as should details of any capital required. If it is shown separately, it will be possible to work out how the practice compares with the average with respect to getting item-of-service payments. Income per patient for a number of items of service is published monthly in *Medeconomics*. It is typical for a new partner to join at half a parity share. This may be negotiable, for instance in the case of older doctors with family commitments, especially if they are moving practice and thus suffering a cut in income.

Working out how your entry in the partnership will affect the profits is a bit more complex:[22]

- Be clear what you are getting a share of. Some practices pool all earnings, but in others PGEA, seniority, outside jobs, training grants etc. are kept by the earner
- Outside jobs and seniority may well be lost with the retiring partner. This will affect profits
- Some expenses may alter when you join, for instance the need to employ locums
- Notional and cost-rent reimbursements may appear in the accounts. If you are not buying in you will not get a share of these, but neither will you bear the loan finance costs
- The accounts will include details of the partners' personal expenses. You will inherit part of these but it takes a few years to build them up to a decent level, and this will affect your tax liability.

The future earning power of the practice is more difficult to predict. A falling list size spells trouble. Overheads tend to stay fixed as you cannot unbuild premises, and sacking staff is not fun.

Tax

Since 1996 each GP has become personally responsible for their own tax liability. Before this all tax was a partnership liability, leading to cases where partners did a runner from the practice without settling their tax bills. All the other financial dealings of the partnership remain the responsibility of the whole partnership.

Capital

All practices have capital assets, even if only fixtures, fittings, drugs, etc. These have to be bought. In addition, all practices need a certain amount of working capital. These are not usually huge sums (unless it is a dispensing practice) and can be covered fairly painlessly.

Since 1965 there have been considerable incentives for GPs to invest in premises under the *Cost-rent scheme*. This is a highly advantageous way of borrowing money, and most GPs do it. However, it does mean that the capital assets of the practice are much higher, and this puts an additional financial burden on the incoming partner.

In general you will be paying off the outgoing partner, and some sort of loan will usually have to be taken out. This will often be done in stages reflecting your current profit share, which is the method most consistent with partnership law. Alternatively, you may not be liable for any of the debt until you reach parity. Another option is that you are not required to purchase any of the partnership assets. This is unusual since the outgoing partner will need to be paid off, and the partnership is likely to work better if all have an interest in its financial health.

The costs of *buying into* the partnership have to be borne at a time when domestic expenditure is likely to be high. You may be moving house, a more reliable or a second car may need to be bought, your spouse may be changing jobs. While you are liable for a part of a partnership debt, you are also entitled to your share of notional or cost-rent reimbursement. Details of the buying-in arrangements should be contained in the partnership deed.

Economic efficiency

A number of parameters of economic efficiency are suggested.[23] Individual practice circumstances may lead to exceptions, but a broad pattern of economic performance can be estimated.

- Total staff costs (before reimbursement) divided by GMS income should be 45 to 50% (and the lower the better)
- Administrative costs (including reimbursements) divided by GMS income should be 9 to 10%
- Professional costs (e.g. accountancy) divided by GMS income should be 2% or less
- Locum costs divided by GMS income should be under 10%
- Fixed income per patient should be more than £24 (£30 in deprived areas)
- Item-of-service income per patient should be more than £10
- Profit per patient – £26 or more
- Staff wages reimbursed: aim for 70%.

The partnership deed

The partnership deed is the written expression of the agreement the partners have with each other. Without one it is impossible to work out whether you are going to be treated fairly by the other partners. This runs the risk that you will suffer abuse, and also means that there is huge potential for disagreement within the practice. Only around half of practices have a written partnership deed. Do not join a practice which has not got a written partnership deed. Model partnership deeds can be obtained from the British Medical Association. Before signing a deed, show it to your solicitor. A deed should include:[24]

- Constitution of the partnership
- Commencement date
- Practice premises and equipment
- Rental or purchase details
- Residential restrictions
- Annual, study and sabbatical leave
- Other absences: maternity, compassionate
- Division of income: private and NHS
- Profit-sharing ratios
- Profits relative to list size
- Liabilities for debts, taxes, gifts
- Accounting procedures
- Banking and accounting details
- Access to practice finances
- Other medical commitments or businesses

- Retirement and expulsion
- Grounds for termination or dissolution.

The common pitfalls

Horror stories are always circulating about how new partners have been misled and abused when joining a practice. Few of these methods of abuse are new, and indeed in some cases merely reflect what was standard practice years ago. Senior partners may be genuinely unaware that their behaviour is unfair, and will be glad to learn that normal practice has changed. In other cases the seniors may be trying to compensate themselves for their own abuse when they joined the practice.

- Check how *parity is defined*. Outside jobs, seniority payments, PGEA etc. may be excluded from the share-out and kept by the individual doctor. Selling goodwill in a medical practice is illegal. If it takes more than three years to get to parity, the partnership may be open to a charge of selling goodwill.[25] Time to parity is now commonly shorter than three years. Some practices pay partners on the basis of their personal list size, which clearly disadvantages the new entrant
- Ensure that there is *parity in workload*. The new partner should not be responsible for more than their fair share of surgeries or on-call duties. If a cooperative or deputising service is used, it should be available to all partners
- Make sure that any *buying-in arrangements are fair*. A way of valuing the practice assets should appear in the partnership deed. It is important that the current market value should be used. For equipment this can be worked out by dividing the purchase cost by the likely life of the equipment, much as is done when claiming depreciation against tax. For premises there may be a conflict of interest where property prices have fallen significantly, especially where notional rent reimbursement has fallen behind the loan repayments
- Look out for *hidden costs*. It was not unusual in past years for the incoming partner to be asked to buy the retiring partner's house, often at an inflated price. Expensive loans or unexpected financial obligations on the practice should be spotted when you show the practice accounts to your accountant
- Be *suspicious* of previous bad practice. If a partner is leaving for reasons other than retirement, try to find out why. Check the health authority records for details of previous partners who have left. It is lucrative for a practice to have a succession of partners who never get to parity. This can be done by forcing partners out of the practice, or by refusing to honour parity agreements.

What if I don't get a job straight away?

Your ideal job is unlikely to be available right away. It is important to have a good look around and see what is available, before making a decision you may have to live with for the next 30 years.

- You will have direct experience of at most two different practices. They are training practices and so not typical

- Retirement vacancies become available when people retire, not just to fit in with the end of the local vocational training scheme.

There are a number of ways to fill any work gaps profitably.

- *Take some time off.* You will probably need a break anyway, and this may be the last chance you have to take prolonged leave
- *Do locum work.* There is plenty available at the moment. This not only plugs the gap, but it also gives you the chance to work in other practices. At the present BMA recommended locum rates it should be possible to get an income approaching what you would expect when joining a partnership. Most GP principals who are appointed have done some locum work beforehand[1]
- Do some more *hospital work.* Some registrars welcome the chance to gain experience in other specialist areas.

Alternatives to being a full-time principal

General practice vocational training traditionally aims at fitting registrars to be full-time principals in general practice. However, more and more newly qualified GPs are opting for alternatives. Even those who join a practice may not regard themselves as committed for more than five years. Alternatives include:

- *Part-time work.* A full-time commitment is 26 hours a week for 42 weeks, three quarter time is 19 hours and half time is 13 hours
- *Non-principal.* Short-term or long-term locum work: a full-timer can get about 75% of a full-time GP principal's pay
- *Deputising service.* Though cooperatives have taken on the bulk of out-of-hours work, deputising agencies still exist to supply locums of all sorts.

Primary Care Act. General practitioner principals have all traditionally been self-employed and have worked according to the *Red Book.* This changed with the NHS (Primary Care) Act of 1997 which gave the option for GPs to work to a much wider variety of contracts. It is now possible for GPs to have their work regulated by a locally agreed contract, as long as that contract fulfils national targets. Under Primary Care Act schemes some GPs have become *employees* (salaried), while others have retained their self-employed status but now work to a different contract. Some health authorities and some general practices are now offering GP jobs on a salaried basis. These jobs tend to be mainly clinical and do not involve the GP in the organisation and finances of the practice. They may also be linked with the achievement of specified local or national care targets.

Other more *innovative* jobs arranged by health authorities have GPs working part-time in primary care and part-time in another specialty such as public health, with perhaps time set aside for continuing professional development or attendance at the local vocational training scheme meetings. These jobs are proving very popular with newly-qualified GPs, many of whom prefer to do the clinical work but not the administrative work of general practice, and who want more time to build up their confidence and experience of medical practice. The jobs are usually time-limited.

- *Job sharing.* Two (or more) GPs share the work of one full-time partner and share the income
- *Other types of general practice.* Work in remote or rural areas, or work in the armed forces, offers different challenges
- *Non-medical.* The achievement of a medical degree involves the acquisition of a lot of skills which have relevance to jobs other than doctoring. However, many will have qualms about such an attitude, having been trained at public expense.

Summary

- The need of the NHS for GPs will probably rise in the future
- Most recently trained GPs do not want to go straight into permanent full-time general practice partnership
- Often the only way to get more details about a job is to make a formal application
- Most jobs in general practice still attract multiple applicants. On being confronted with a lot of CVs and covering letters, many practices will first look for ways of excluding some or most of the applications. The primary task of an application is to be noticed and not discarded
- The average GP is much more concerned about money than is the average registrar
- Getting a job in general practice is not like winning a raffle. You and the job must match. It helps nobody if a partnership breaks down
- You are interviewing your future partners just as much as they are interviewing you
- If fully implemented, the NHS (Primary Care) Act will make profound changes in how primary care is organised in the future
- Any practice which does not have a practice agreement (partnership deed) cannot regulate its internal business properly and so is to be avoided.

Topics for discussion

- A job in general practice is for life
- The *Red Book* (Statement of Fees and Allowances) and the present GP contract are holding back the development of primary care
- Work as a non-principal should only be temporary
- GPs should look for the jobs where they are most needed
- In the selection of a partner, only the best person will get the job.

References

1. Handysides S. Returning to general practice. BMJ Classified 20 January 2001: 2–3.
2. Anon. Number of part-timers grows. *General Practitioner* December 4 1998: 3.
3. *Medeconomics* 2001; 22(6) June.
4. Allen I. Career preferences of doctors. *BMJ* 1996; 313: 2.
5. Anon. GP numbers rise and fall in the UK. *General Practitioner* February 9 2001: 14.

6. Briefing. *BMJ* Classified 11 March 2000: 3.
7. Hartley J. Largest fall in joiners in a decade. *General Practitioner* June 2 2000: 26.
8. Ebdy M. Where are all the trainees? *Medical Monitor* 1996; 9(10): 22.
9. Pownall M. Workforce timebomb. *Best Practice* 14 February 2001: 12.
10. Davies J. GP recruitment tops pay agenda. *Medeconomics* 1997; 18(10): 45–6.
11. Thomson R. Are you one of the new breed of GPs? *Medeconomics* 1993; 14(12): 62–3.
12. Laws C. I don't want to be a GP. *Medeconomics* 1994; 15(5): 73–81.
13. Beardow R, Cheung K and Styles W McN. Factors influencing the career choices of general practitioner trainees in North West Thames Regional Health Authority. *Br J Gen Pract* 1993; 43: 449–52.
14. Vincent P. Choosing a practice. *Update* 1993; 47: 52–5.
15. Thomson R. Do your homework before you buy in. *Medeconomics* 1994; 15(1): 57–8.
16. North M A. Evaluation of the experience of trainees seeking employment after completion of their vocational training. *J Roy Coll Gen Pract.* 1985; 35: 29–33.
17. Roberts J (ed). Curriculum Vitae. *Pulse 'in practice'.* January 21 1989: 77–82.
18. Gray R. The perfect graduate CV. *Cosmopolitan,* June 1993: 133–5.
19. Khunti K. Applying for a partnership. *Update* 1993; 47: 304–7.
20. Fisher P. *Guardian* 4 February 1995.
21. Munson S. Interview Checklist. *Medeconomics* 1993; 14(7): 49.
22. Slavin S. Assess the earning power of your new practice. *Medeconomics* 1993; 14(2): 96.
23. Slavin L. How to assess financial performance. *General Practitioner* March 31 2000: 70.
24. Clayson M. Becoming a practice principal. *The Practitioner* 1994; 238: 270–3.
25. Dean J. What to watch out for when choosing your practice. *Monitor Weekly* 1994; 7(11): 57–9.

Getting patients to take their medicines

Tutorial aim	**The registrar can issue prescriptions which patients are likely to take properly.**
Learning objectives	By the end of the tutorial the registrar can: • Give four reasons why patients may not take their medicines properly • List five general ways to improve medicine-taking by patients • List three ways to improve medicine-taking in the elderly • Give two reasons why patients should take their medicines properly • Discuss the implications of inaccurate drug taking • Discuss the limitations of prescribing in disease • Help a patient achieve a medication regimen which is likely to be taken accurately.

Introduction

Prescribing medication to a patient is restricted in the United Kingdom to practitioners named in the Medical Register. It is one of over 700 privileges of registration, but is probably the one over which GPs spend most time and effort. However the simple issuing of a prescription, whether it is for an effective remedy or not, is only part of a doctor's obligation towards a patient. The likelihood is that the medication will not be used as intended. This is not surprising. Many recommendations which doctors make to patients have little or no effect: for example, the effectiveness of GPs in altering patients' lifestyle habits is disappointing at best, and at worst a complete waste of breath.

The word *compliance* was for many years applied to the problem of patients who will not take their pills properly. The rules were clear: the doctor's job was to prescribe the right pills, and the patient's job was to take them as instructed. This represents a rather doctor-centred and paternalistic view of doctor-patient interactions. People are rational within their own terms. If a patient does not agree with a doctor about a management plan, then it is unusual for that plan to be challenged openly since most patients do not have the knowledge or confidence to mount such a challenge. It is more likely that patients will vote with their feet and express their unhappiness by not taking their treatment as prescribed. The word *compliance* infers that the patient's role is passive and submissive, when this is far from being true. The Royal Pharmaceutical Society of Great Britain (who, among their other work, are joint publishers with the BMA of the British National Formulary) prefer the term *concordance* which emphasises that fact that if doctor and patient are able to see eye to eye about a prescribed treatment, then that treatment is much more likely to be taken properly.

For the *drug manufacturer* also the stakes are high. If a treatment is effective but patients for some reason will not take it, then the treatment will not succeed and doctors will not prescribe it. In these cases the manufacturer will be tempted to blame the patient rather than the product for treatment failure. Compliance, with its authoritarian overtones, implies a certain contempt for patients who will not do as they are told and take their medicine.

The context

British general practitioners are very keen on medicines.

- In 1995 GPs wrote prescriptions for over 470 million items at a total cost of over £3 600 million, or 10% of the entire NHS budget;[1] while in 1999 the cost of prescriptions issued by GPs and dentists was £5.3 billion[1]
- The number of prescribed items per person is continuing to rise, and the overall cost of drugs to the NHS rises well ahead of inflation[2]
- A prescription is issued during around 65% of all GP consultations, and at any one time 40% of the population is taking a prescribed medicine[3]
- Three quarters of items, and four fifths in terms of cost of all prescribed medications, are given on repeat so that the patient is not seen at the time.[4]

In fact, GPs are rather keener on medicines than are their patients.

- In one study, 51% of patients went into their consultation with the GP expecting to be given a prescription, but 55% actually received one[5]
- Many patients show a distinct preference for avoiding medication especially in some sorts of illness. For example it is probable that a majority of cases of major depression can be helped by medication, and that counselling is relatively ineffective. However, less than half of the general population think antidepressants are effective, but 85% think that counselling works.[6]

Anything between 5[7] and 20%[8] of prescriptions never get as far as the pharmacist.

- Some patients do not like taking medicines at all, but are reluctant to tell their doctor
- Others do not agree with the proposed treatment because they are unhappy with something that happened in the consultation[9]
- Yet others cannot afford the prescription charges[10]
- Undoubtedly, some prescriptions just get lost: the common practice of post-dating prescriptions for oral contraceptives contributes to 25% of these never being dispensed.[11]

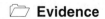 **Evidence**

Reasons for not having prescriptions dispensed[12]

A small study from general practice of uncashed prescriptions found that reasons given by patients for their behaviour included:[12]

- Cheaper over the counter (drug obtained), 41%
- Deterred by cost, 23%
- Doctor's 'permission' not to cash the prescription
- Poor understanding of the illness
- A wish to retain control.

Even if the prescription is dispensed, there is no guarantee that the medicine will be taken at all. Some patients on long-term medication will attend their doctor regularly for review of their condition, get the prescription dispensed, and then either throw the medicine away or more often hoard it. The psychological mechanism of such behaviour is complex,[7] but denial may play a part. The patient may have a desire to outwit the illness or the GP. Most GPs will have an anecdote or two, told against themselves and their hospital colleagues, about patients who hoard unused medication. The more spectacular cases even reach the medical journals, such as the report in the British Medical Journal on the 80-year-old lady whose family, after her death, returned 278 items weighing 6 kg, stockpiled over five years.[4]

For those patients who do take their medicine, *nearly all of them do not take it as prescribed*.

- Studies in children taking penicillin have shown that by day three only 46% have penicillin present in the urine, and by day six this has fallen to 31%[9]
- There is less incentive to take medicine when acute symptoms have abated. It is estimated that *half* of patients take their medicines *sufficiently accurately* to achieve therapeutic objectives, and the other half do not.[13]

Long-term treatments tend to be taken more accurately.[14] Even so, one study of people taking beta blockers for hypertension and angina found that 20% took the tablets as prescribed, 46% took between 80 and 120% of the dose and some took up to twice the prescribed dose.[9] If these figures are to be believed, *unintentional overdose* may be as big a problem as under-treatment. Some patients will take a periodic *drug holiday* from their treatment, thus running the risks of decreased effectiveness and also of withdrawal effects which may be interpreted as a new illness. In the relatively common *white coat adherence* a patient may take medication properly only during the week or so before attending the doctor.[15]

Does it matter?

Improved outcomes

If a medication is taken according to the manufacturer's recommendations it is more likely to be effective. A licence is granted to a medicine only when trials have confirmed that it does what it is supposed to do. The licence includes details of the conditions for which the licence is valid and for the doses of treatment to be used. Subjects in a drug trial are subjects because they have consciously agreed to be involved. They are also likely to be under close review during the trial. Accordingly it is probable that subjects in a drug trial are more likely to take their medications in the right dose and at the right time when compared to the more autonomous individuals who might be prescribed the same drug after the trials are completed and when it becomes available for wider prescription. Accordingly, the granting of a product licence to a drug is based on the evidence of clinical trials using people who have taken the drug in accordance with the licence. Patients who do not take their medicines as accurately are therefore less likely to get the full benefits of their medicines. It is estimated that attempts to reduce the risk of heart attacks and stroke would be up to twice as effective if patients took their antihypertensive medicine properly.[13]

Previous experiences

The experiences which people have with episodes of illness and the taking of medication will affect their concordance with medical advice. In a logical world, ill people would take their medicine and get better. This is only one of four possible scenarios:[16]

- The patient takes the medicine and gets better. Taking the medicine was clearly the right thing to do. Both patient and GP are happy with their decisions
- The patient does not take the medicine, or takes the medicine incorrectly, and does not get better. The patient has been insubordinate and is suffering the consequences
- The patient takes the medicine and does not get better. Either the diagnosis is wrong or the treatment is wrong: either way the GP is a fool and not to be trusted further
- The patient does not take the medicine and gets better. This is not disastrous for the patient, except that a prescription charge may have been levied. However, it makes the prescriber look rather silly.

Limitations to prescribing

There are a number of reasons other than the cussedness of patients why treatment will not bring about the expected results, even if concordance is adequate.

- As most GPs will admit, prescribing has an element of *guesswork* about it. The prescriber cannot be sure that a sore throat will respond to penicillin. On clinical appearance alone it is impossible to judge which sore throats have a bacterial cause, and even if bacteria are present their antibiotic sensitivity can only be guessed at. Waiting for the throat swab result leads to an unacceptable delay in treatment
- If a prescription is not issued at all, then there is no medication regimen to comply with or otherwise. Different doctors have *different prescribing practices*. One doctor's bronchitis is another doctor's viral chest infection. On Friday evenings before a bank holiday, GPs are probably more likely

to prescribe antibiotics. Prescribing sometimes also reflects national practice: for example, it is normal in Holland to treat otitis media with analgesia and surveillance, whereas in Britain sufferers are more likely to be prescribed antibiotics

- Many medicines are prescribed as a *therapeutic trial* to confirm the diagnosis and help the patient at the same time
- Other medicines are purely *symptomatic* and so buy time for the illness to cure itself.

The prescribing of medicine may not be the best way to treat the condition: one small study from general practice found that for illnesses with symptoms but no signs, the positive attitude of the practitioner had more effect than whether or not medicine was prescribed.[17]

Improving concordance

When medicine is prescribed, there is a three-way interaction between the medicine, the patient and the doctor. The doctor is the professional, and so has the responsibility to help the patient to take the medicine at least to the extent that it is likely to do some good. It is almost impossible to predict which patients will or will not take their medicines adequately.[8] However, there are techniques which are known to help.

Satisfaction

Patient satisfaction is a legitimate aim of medical practice, not only because it ensures better relations between doctors and patients, but also because *health outcomes are likely to be improved*. Patients who are more satisfied with a consultation are more likely to follow the advice given.[16] That satisfaction should affect concordance is quite plausible. All patients will enter a consultation with *ideas* about their symptoms and what should be done about them. If the doctor fails to agree with those ideas or does not offer a believable alternative, then the patient may well feel that they have been unable to communicate their problem properly. Some patients are assertive enough to tell their doctor if they do not feel they have had a decent hearing. Most of the others can only register their frustration by declining to follow the advice offered. If patients cannot agree with the diagnosis, they are unlikely to take the treatment seriously.

📄 Guidelines

Improving patient satisfaction[18]

Increased information given by doctor
Technical and interpersonal competence
Partnership building (see next box)
Positive talk
Positive non-verbal behaviour
Social conversation
Talk calm but behave concerned.

Doctors also have a need to feel satisfied by a consultation. A doctor may be prompted to prescribe because of a desire to maintain the doctor-patient relationship rather than a positive belief that the prescription will help. A study from South Wales of prescribing for sore throat revealed that the GPs involved felt uncomfortable when prescribing antibiotics against the evidence, but that did not stop them. Interestingly, patient satisfaction did not seem to be influenced much by the prescribing or otherwise of an antibiotic. Explanations of the differences between viruses and bacteria were held to be confusing, and mothers were happier to accept non-antibiotic treatment for their children than they were for themselves. Many wished *further information and pain relief.*[19]

Health beliefs

Achieving patient satisfaction requires that the GP finds out what the patient's beliefs are, and tailors any advice to be consistent with them. This is part of partnership building.

📄 **Guidelines**

Partnership building with patients

Patients are more content when[16]

- the doctor discovers and attends to their concerns and expectations
- communicates warmth, interest and concern
- explains matters in terms which the patient can understand.

Patients follow treatment more closely when they believe they can have some control over their health.[16] Health beliefs can be readily altered by discussion with a doctor. Patients, being rational, will gladly change their minds if the alternative presented is plausible.

- Patients are more likely to take their medicines if they think it will do them some good
- Where a medicine improves a symptom it is easier to understand that the medicine is beneficial
- Where a medicine is supposed to avert the complications of an illness, such as the use of medicine in hypertension to prevent stroke, then a patient is influenced by how vulnerable they feel or how likely they think it is that they will suffer the complication. This *perceived vulnerability* is most readily influenced by *anecdote*, such as whether a friend or family member has suffered such a complication,[9] but discussion with the GP will also have some effect
- *Side effects* will put patients off taking their treatment properly, especially if the side effects are not mentioned in advance
- Many people have *specific beliefs* about medicines[13]

   they are unnatural
   they are addictive
   they are intrinsically dangerous
   the beneficial effects will decrease.

Drug formulation

It is self-evident that patients are less likely to take their medicines if they do not taste nice or if they are hard to swallow. Some patients can tolerate tablets but not capsules or vice versa. Most children prefer liquids. To the person with arthritic hands childproof containers may also be adultproof. Patients who cannot read the labels on the medicines are unlikely to be able to take them accurately.[20]

Regimen complexity

The more medicines prescribed, the less likely it is that they will be taken as prescribed. In the elderly, in whom polypharmacy is common, poor concordance is more likely.[13] Good practice requires a regular review of medication: when a new drug is introduced, it is helpful if an old one can be discarded. The Royal College of Physicians recommends that the elderly should not be required to take more than four different medications on a regular basis.[15] The chance of an adverse event due to medication increases with the complexity of the regimen[21] and also with the number of different drugs in use. This is a particular problem for the elderly, and should be considered when each new symptom is being tackled with a new medication.

Patients find it equally *easy to take one or two doses* of medication a day. Beyond this the chance of concordance falls.[9] Modified release products and combination products may not provide the economy and flexibility of the unmodified drug, but if they are more likely to be taken properly then the extra expense is justified. If a little forethought is not applied, it is quite possible for a patient to end up on a drug regimen where some medicines are taken four times a day, some three times, some with meals, some on an empty stomach, and some where the instructions on the label are inadequate. Such a regimen is virtually impossible to follow.

If the drug routine does not fit with the patient's *daily routine* it is unlikely to be followed. What is a patient to do when faced with four times a day dosage with meals if only three meals a day are eaten? What is a night worker to do with the night dosage, especially on days off? Does three times a day mean every eight hours, or three during daytime? You may want your patient to take their antibiotic round the clock, but their nitrate only by day.

Feedback

Getting a patient involved in monitoring their condition will improve concordance.[9] This is particularly useful where treatment is prolonged but the effects of treatment are not obvious from a change in symptoms. The self-monitoring of blood glucose in diabetics is now quite normal, and more hypertensives are buying their own measuring equipment.

Information

Offering information is generally a good way of improving patient satisfaction with a consultation. Information may be welcomed about all aspects of the condition being treated, not just those related to any medication being prescribed.

- Only around 7% of consultation time is spent in GPs telling patients about their treatment[7]
- Leaflets are handed out by GPs to around one in five patients,[22] favouring the higher social classes

- Fifty-four per cent of patients want comprehensive information about their medicines, and a further 43% want short, snappy points.[23]

📁 **Evidence**

> **Patient information needs[23]**
>
> A study from Southampton identified seven items of drug information which were felt by patients to be important:
>
> - When and how to take the medicine
> - Unwanted effects and what to do about them
> - Precautions, such as possible effects on driving
> - Problems with alcohol or other drugs
> - The name of the medicine
> - The purpose of the treatment
> - What to do if a dose is missed.

Under EC directive 89/341 many of these points are now required to be included on a user leaflet inserted into the manufacturer's packs of medication,[22] but this will only be received by a patient when an *original pack* is dispensed. Specimens of the leaflets have been circulated to doctors by the Association of the British Pharmaceutical Industry in the form of a compendium.

Patient problems

Patients who have *chronic illness* and who are also *depressed* are three times more likely not to take their medication accurately than are patients who are physically ill but psychologically well.[24] It is not clear if the depression is a cause of or a consequence of the poor concordance.

People who are less likely to take their medicines properly include[15]

- The elderly
- The mentally ill
- Ethnic minorities.

Inducements

In work on the treatment of tuberculosis, where poor concordance with prolonged courses of drugs has resulted in drug resistance problems, various methods have been tried to induce patients to stick to their treatments properly. Interventions of proven effectiveness are:[25]

- Reminder cards
- Help from lay health workers
- Monetary incentives
- Health education
- Combined health education and monetary incentives
- Close supervision.

The most effective strategy is education plus payment. Interestingly there are no plans by the government to make payments to patients who take their tablets more accurately.

If all else fails

For some patients complex drug regimens are inevitable, and for others even following simplified regimens is very difficult. In these cases, medication can be given by a *carer* or a professional. Depot injections can be useful particularly in chronic schizophrenia. Hospitalising tuberculosis patients improves their uptake of medication significantly. More sneaky methods of checking up on patients include testing the urine for drug metabolites, or putting chemical markers in the medication. Bottle-tops with microchips can tell you when the bottle has been opened.

In the NOMAD scheme, the pharmacist lays out all the patient's medication in a compartmentalised tray, and then seals the top with clear plastic. The patient or carer can tell at a glance what medication has been taken. There is however no deterrent for the patient who wishes to take more than their prescribed dose.

Epilogue

The medicine is not an end in itself: the restoring to health of the patient is what is important. It does not really matter to the GP what the patient does with the medicine as long as the outcome is beneficial. Such was the faith of some ancient Chinese patients in their doctor that it was considered adequate to eat the paper the prescription was written on in order to cure the illness: now there was real authority.

Summary

- Doctors are keener on drug treatments than patients are
- Nearly all patients take their medicines in contravention of medical advice
- Around half of patients take their medicines accurately enough for them to do some good
- A minority of patients will not take drugs at all, usually without telling the prescriber
- A patient who agrees with a proposed management is more likely to take their medicine more accurately
- Prescribing in general practice is often incompletely scientific
- Improving patient satisfaction with a consultation improves the likelihood of any medicine being taken properly
- Some patient groups have particular difficulty taking medicines accurately
- The elderly tend to be submitted to complex drug regimens. Try to keep to a maximum of four drugs, each with one or two doses a day
- Most patients want to know more about their medicines than they are told.

🗩 Topics for discussion

- Patients who do not take their medicines properly must accept the consequences
- Suggest a management plan for:

    A school-age child with tonsillitis
    An elderly widow with an itchy rash on her back
    A shift worker with depression
    An elderly man with angina, heart failure and osteoarthritis

A demented woman whose daughter brings in two carrier bags of untaken medication.

References

1. Prescription costs are slowing down. *General Practitioner* August 2 1996: Hartley J. *General Practitioner* July 21 2000: 12.
2. Anon. England's drug bill rises. *In Brief. BMJ* 2000; 321: 468.
3. George C F. Introducing PILS. *MIMS Magazine* 1988; 15: 75–80.
4. Minerva. *BMJ* 1999; 318: 1018.
5. Webb S and Lloyd M. Prescribing and referral in general practice: a study of patients' expectations and doctors' actions. *Br J Gen Pract* 1994; 44: 165–9.
6. Market and Opinion Research International poll. Attitudes towards depression. London: Royal College of Psychiatrists, 1992.
7. Knox J D E. The five elements that make for non-compliance. *Modern Medicine* 1989; 34: 391–4.
8. Aronson J K and Hardman M. Patient compliance. *BMJ* 1992; 305: 1009–11.
9. George C F. How to get your patients to take their medicine. *Update* 1994: 48: 518–23.
10. Waters A. Scrip charges deter one-in-five from GP. *General Practitioner* July 7 1995: 10.
11. Bearden P H G, McGilchrist M M, McKendrick A D et al. Primary non-compliance with prescribed medication in primary care. *BMJ* 1993; 307: 846–8.
12. Jones I and Britten N. Why do some patients not cash their prescriptions? *Br J Gen Pract* 1998; 48: 903–5.
13. Bradley C. Compliance with drug therapy. *Prescribers' Journal* 1999; 39(1): 44–50.
14. Haines P. One quarter of drug courses unfinished. *General Practitioner* February 2 1996: 28.
15. Thistlethwaite J. Compliance problems in practice. Training *Update* June 1998: 6–9.
16. Pendleton D, Schofield T, Tate P and Havelock P. The Consultation. Oxford: Oxford University Press, 1994.
17. Thomas K B. General practice consultations: is there any point in being positive? *BMJ* 1984; 294: 1200–02.
18. Silverman J, Kurtz S and Draper J. Skills for Communicating with Patients. Abingdon: Radcliffe, 1998.
19. Butler C C, Rollnick S, Pill R *et al*. Understanding the culture of prescribing: a qualitative study of general practitioners' and patients' perceptions of antibiotics for sore throats. *BMJ* 1998; 317: 637–42.
20. Reilly H. Confident patients will take medicine. *General Practitioner* November 11 1994: 6.
21. Pearson T. Complex medical problems increase the rate of adverse effects in the elderly. *Medical Monitor* 10 May 2000: 33.
22. Greenhalgh T. User leaflets. *BMJ* 1990; 300: 420–1.
23. George C F. What do patients need to know about prescribed drugs? *Prescribers' Journal* 1994; 34(1): 7–11.
24. Minerva. *BMJ* 2000; 321: 460.
25. Volmink J and Garner P. Systematic review of randomised controlled trials of strategies to promote adherence to tuberculosis treatment. *BMJ* 1997; 315: 1403–6.

Headache

Tutorial aim	**The registrar should be able to manage at least 80% of patients with headache presenting in general practice.**
Learning objectives	By the end of the tutorial the registrar can: • Recall four diagnostic features of migraine • Recall two treatments for acute migraine and three prophylactic treatments for migraine • Discuss the avoidance of migraine triggers • Recall three diagnostic features of tension headache • Discuss with a patient the causes and treatments of tension headache • Choose a management option for tension headache • Discuss the effects of headache on life • Describe a suitable clinical examination for headache • Refer to hospital appropriately, with appropriate urgency.

How common is headache?

- Nearly 90% of all people have headache in a given year[1]
- Over any two-week period, 25% of the population will have a headache severe enough to take an analgesic; 10% will have at least one very severe headache each year[2]
- Between 1% and 2% of sufferers will present themselves to their GP with their symptoms.[2]

🗀 **Evidence**

> **Prevalence of headache[3]**
>
> A telephone survey in America found that 5% of adult women and almost 3% of men had more than 180 headaches a year.

Headaches are either *primary*, or *secondary* to an underlying cause. Tension causes about 70% of primary headaches, and migraine another 15%. In over 60% of cases, secondary headache is caused by systemic *infection* and pyrexia.[4]

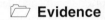 **Evidence**

> ### Diagnoses of headache in general practice[5]
>
> Patients consulting their GP because of headache
>
> - 40% tension headache
> - 30% migraine
> - 30% other diagnoses
> - children aged 5 to 15, migraine is commoner[6]
> - children with headache tend to become adults with recurring headache.[7]

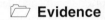 **Evidence**

> ### Diagnoses of headache in secondary care[2]
>
> Around 20% of consulters will be referred to hospital, and headache accounts for 25% of all neurology referrals. The results of these referrals
>
> - 3% tumour
> - 5% other serious cause
> - 70% benign cause of headache
> - 22% no diagnosis.

The social cost of headache can be considerable. For instance it was estimated (1999) that migraine costs the UK nearly £2 billion a year, less than a tenth of which is medical costs.[8]

Serious causes of headache

For each person who presents to their GP with headache, less than 2% will have serious underlying pathology.[9] On average a GP will see a new brain tumour only once every 10 years. It is nonetheless important not to miss serious pathology when it does arise, and much of the routine assessment of headache is directed at excluding serious disease.

Raised intracranial pressure

Headache is usually a *late symptom* of raised intracranial pressure,[10] and so there will nearly always be other symptoms or signs.

- Headache starts gradually and progressively worsens
- Pain is poorly localised and worse on lying down, coughing and stooping
- Typically begins early in the morning and wakes the patient from sleep
- Examination may reveal focal neurological signs or altered consciousness and papilloedema.

Brain tumour is commonest in the over-55s. However in the rare instance of a childhood tumour, headache, vomiting and ataxia or unsteadiness are particularly worrying features.

Meningitis

Bacterial meningitis is characterised by:

- Throbbing headache

- Systemic disturbance with fever, photophobia, neck stiffness
- Altered consciousness.

Urgent administration of phenoxymethyl penicillin and admission to hospital is needed and may be life saving. Viral meningitis tends to run a milder course. *Encephalitis* may cause headache, but there is also evidence of cerebral dysfunction with confusion, clouding of consciousness and disorientation.

Haemorrhage

Subarachnoid haemorrhage (SAH) usually presents very acutely and is often described by those who are able to do so as like being hit very hard on the back of the head. Sudden loss of consciousness often results and death is not infrequent. Patients most likely to benefit from surgery are those with a severe headache but no other symptoms, i.e. those in whom the diagnosis of SAH is most likely to be missed.[11] Up to 60% of cases are preceded by one or a number of *warning leaks* in the month before the haemorrhage.[12] In these episodes a severe headache occurs with pain in the head or face which is often hemicranial, hemifacial or periorbital. A third nerve palsy may occur, as may vomiting and photophobia. The presence of neck stiffness is particularly significant.

The *elderly brain* is particularly sensitive to trauma, however slight, because of brain shrinkage. *Extra-dural haemorrhage* is usually caused by a bleed from the middle meningeal artery. After a head injury all is apparently well for several hours (the *lucid interval*) until the rapid onset of a deteriorating level of consciousness. In subdural haemorrhage the preceding trauma may be minor and forgotten. Several days later the bleed expresses itself as headache, a fluctuating level of consciousness and sometimes personality changes.

Giant cell (temporal) arteritis

This affects older patients and is often associated with polymyalgia rheumatica. There is a temporal headache of a persistent nature which traditionally comes to light when patients are afflicted when putting on a hat or brushing their hair. Localised *scalp tenderness* and sometimes a cord-like and very tender cranial artery may be palpated. An *ESR over 50 mm/h* is typical[1] but not universal, and though a cranial artery biopsy may confirm the diagnosis it is only 60 to 70% sensitive.[13] The most important complication is of sudden permanent *blindness* if the retinal artery becomes involved. Early treatment with steroids is required.

Tension headache

Tension headache is by far the *commonest type of primary headache*, and is five times commoner than migraine.[1] Most tension headaches are not presented to a doctor, but even so a GP with a list of 2000 can expect four or five new cases to present each year.[14] The headaches may be episodic or chronic, often having been present for months or years. Typically the pain is described as a *weight on the head* or a *tight band round the head*. There may be associated nausea, photophobia and phonophobia, but vomiting is rare. Despite the vivid language with which the sufferers may describe their headaches, *normal activities are usually unimpaired*. Indeed exertion or regular more gentle exercise often improves the symptoms. Physical signs are usually absent. In some cases the neck and shoulder muscles show increased tone.

Some sufferers will have symptoms of depression or anxiety, the treatment of which will help the headaches. Some will have been subject to recent emotional stress: identification of such stress can make a diagnosis of tension more acceptable.

Aetiology The cause of tension headache is *unknown*. Emotional, psychological and muscular causes have been suggested.[15] Since not every case is the headache due to tension, it is proposed to use the alternative term *tension-type headache*.[15]

It may prove difficult to convince a patient with tension headache that psychological illness can cause physical symptoms. Pain is usually associated with tissue damage, and analgesia simply masks the symptom without addressing the underlying cause. It is hard to believe that the pain does not represent some physical disorder. It is easier to understand that *muscle overuse can cause pain*, which is why arms ache after carrying heavy shopping. Neck muscle ache can radiate over the scalp and cause headache. Such an explanation of tension headache may not be strictly true, but it is certainly *plausible* and emphasises the essentially benign nature of the headache.

Tension headache has traditionally been regarded as a dustbin in which to deposit headaches for which it has not been possible to find a more medically interesting cause. Such a diagnosis of exclusion may partially satisfy the practitioner but is unlikely to convince the sufferers, who are more interested in what they have got rather than what they have not got. Dissatisfied patients are less likely to comply with medical advice and less likely to get better. The effective GP will make efforts to reach a *positive diagnosis* of tension headache, and offer a plausible explanation to the patient.

Treatment Treatment response is *often disappointing*, one diagnostic pointer being that *simple analgesia is often only partially effective* despite full dosage, and stronger analgesics confer little additional benefit. Indeed the use of analgesics may actually make the headache worse. If analgesics in the mild narcotic class (e.g. codeine) or ergotamine are taken over the course of three months or more at a rate of more than three times a week[16] or more than 30 tablets a month, a headache may be caused which then only temporarily resolves with the next dose of medication – *Analgesic headache*.

Increasing levels of *exercise* may help. A psychological approach, possibly including psychotherapy, counselling and emotional support may also help, but there is little supportive evidence for these treatments in headache.[15] Some patients will *not take kindly* to suggestions that their pain is psychosomatic: this will be taken as an inference that the pain is imaginary.

- *Non-steroidal anti-inflammatory agents* may help the headache more than simple analgesics
- In chronic tension headache *amitriptyline* (but not other antidepressants) has been shown to have a benefit separate from any antidepressant activity.

The starting dose is 10 mg a day, building to a maximum of 100 mg a day.[15] Not a licensed use

- *Propranolol* 30 mg to 120 mg a day may also help. Not a licensed use
- Where available, *biofeedback*, behavioural programmes and relaxation are worth a try.[17]

It is usually not possible to cure tension headache. Treatment may however reduce the frequency and severity of episodes.

Tension headache and migraine can coexist, a situation which used to be called *combination headache*. Treatment should be directed towards the most important headache for the patient, but migraine is usually easier to treat.

Migraine

- Typically the first attack occurs during the *teens or early twenties*. It is rare for a first attack of migraine to occur over the age of 50,[17] though it is not uncommon for attacks to recur into the 40s
- On average each migraine sufferer gets one attack per month.[17] The attacks often abate during middle age, but there is always a chance that the symptoms will restart
- The peak age for attacks is 20 to 40.[5]

Migraine often causes more symptoms than just headache. For each sufferer the pattern of *each attack is more or less the same*. Indeed if there is a change in the pattern of the symptoms it is important to make a fresh assessment to find out if there is another cause for the headaches. The migraine sufferer is quite well between attacks, however severe they are. If the unwellness is persisting, this again casts doubt on the diagnosis.

🗁 Evidence

How common is Migraine?[16]	
Lifetime incidence	8% of men and 25% of women
Prevalence	12%
Self-treating	70%
Under continuing medical care	3%

The *prodrome* occurs for about a *day* before the headache, and causes subtle changes in mood or behaviour. There may be lethargy and yawning, or sometimes a feeling of extreme well-being. There may be insatiable hunger and cravings.

The *aura* consists of neurological symptoms which occur in the *hour* or so before the headache starts. Visual symptoms may include the highly characteristic *fortification spectra* where objects appear to have battlement-shaped edges. Alternatively there may be *focal motor or sensory symptoms* which may be very similar to those you might expect to follow a stroke. Such symptoms can be particularly alarming. Virtually all patients with aura have visual symptoms, a third have sensory symptoms, two thirds have motor symptoms and a fifth have trouble talking.[18]

The *headache* of migraine is typically severe and throbbing, and lasts from *4 to 72 hours*. It is accompanied by nausea or vomiting and photophobia. The pain may occur all over the head but *typically is localised* to just one part, usually a hemisphere.

Types of Migraine In 1988 the *International Headache Society* published diagnostic criteria for migraine.[4] Migraine treatment can only hope to work if the diagnosis is correct in the first place.

- *Migraine with aura* (formerly called classical migraine, 25% of cases[19]). The aura can last up to 60 minutes, and symptoms resolve completely. Headache follows within an hour of the aura[20]
- *Migraine without aura* (formerly called common migraine). The headache lasts between four and 72 hours and is associated with one or more of:[20]

    Nausea
    Photophobia
    Phonophobia

- The *headache* must also show two or more of these features:

    Unilateral
    Pulsating
    Moderate to severe intensity
    Aggravated by movement

- *Hemiplegic (focal) migraine*: the aura includes focal neurological symptoms
- *Complicated migraine*: neurological signs persist after the acute attack
- *Cluster headache*: see next section.

The acute migraine attack

Aspirin 900 mg (3 tablets) is the first choice for the acute attack.[19] Paracetamol 1000 mg (2 tablets) can be used in the aspirin-sensitive. *Non-steroidal anti-inflammatory agents* can also be used, but most are not licensed for this indication: some are available as suppositories, which is useful if vomiting is a problem. Stronger analgesics rarely offer additional benefits,[16] and opioids are best avoided.[19] Gastric stasis is a feature of migraine. *Soluble analgesia* therefore works better,[21] and tablets should be taken with food as early as possible in the attack. The addition of metoclopramide or domperidone eases nausea or vomiting and improves the analgesic effect. *Soluble aspirin 900 mg plus metoclopramide 10 mg* improves headache in up to half of migraine attacks.[19]

Oral triptans can be used as a second line. They are better tolerated than aspirin/metoclopramide, but no more effective for pain and less good for nausea.[19] Sumatriptan 100 mg costs £8 a tablet (compared with 3.3p for aspirin 900 mg and metoclopramide 10 mg). It is also available as a nasal spray (£6 a dose) and a subcutaneous injection (£20.57 a dose), and these are the preparations of choice if the migraine is causing vomiting[19] (1998 prices). Most people with migraine want to *sleep*, and this often helps.

Most *proprietary treatments* for migraine are combinations of a simple analgesic and an anti-emetic, and many are available without prescription. If prescribed they attract only one prescription charge, but the doses of the different components cannot be titrated for the individual patient.

Avoiding triggers

Up to *50%* of patients can help themselves by avoiding situations in which their migraine is likely to occur.[16] The link can be established by the use of a *migraine diary* where over a period of time the patient records any factors which might trigger an attack, and the pattern of the attacks. The migraine process starts *up to two days* before the headache emerges, so the timing of the trigger has to be noted. Different triggers may be relevant in different migraine sufferers.[22] They are *cumulative*, so that one or more triggers may increase the risk of an attack to a threshold beyond which an attack results. Examples include:

- Insufficient food, missing meals, delayed meals
- Specific foods are responsible in 20% of cases[10]
- Emotional stress and overwork
- Sleep: too little or too much
- Environmental triggers such as bright lights, overexertion, weather
- Hormonal triggers such as the oral contraceptive or hormone replacement therapy. If migraine with focal neurological symptoms occurs for the first time in somebody taking a combined oral contraceptive pill, this should be discontinued. Even migraine without focal neurological signs has been associated with an increased risk of stroke.[23]

Migraine prophylaxis

Some (but not all) sufferers will prefer to try to avoid migraine attacks. Attacks are at best disabling and at worst alarming. Treatment of an acute attack takes time and may be incompletely effective. Prophylaxis should be offered where there are *more than two attacks a month,*[19] or if the patient requests it.

Prophylactic medication should be *tried for three to six months*, and then the situation re-assessed.

- *Propranolol* 10 mg to 120 mg a day is first choice, and reduces the frequency, duration and intensity of migraine attacks by *nearly half.*[19] The benefits may wear off with time, but restarting the drug later may work
- *Pizotifen* 0.5 mg to 4.5 mg a day will help some migraine sufferers, but troublesome *side effects* (sedation, weight gain) are common[19]
- *Tricyclic antidepressants*[17] (but not SSRIs) are useful
- *Sodium valproate* also works, but does not have a licence[19]
- *Clonidine* has a licence for migraine prophylaxis, but it *does not work*[20]
- *Calcium-channel blockers* are used in many parts of the world, but are not licensed for use for migraine in the UK. They are about as effective as propranolol
- *Feverfew* (Tanacetum parthenium) is a herbal remedy which is effective, possibly because of antiprostaglandin activity. It may cause a sore tongue, dyspepsia and mouth ulcers
- *Homeopathy* and/or *acupuncture* may be effective in some cases. They are

probably effective but have not as yet been submitted to formal clinical evaluation[10]

- An *aspirin a day* may work in some patients.

Exotic headaches

Other headaches are occasionally encountered by the GP.[17] Many are quite dramatic in their presentation.

Cluster headaches are very severe unilateral head pains, occurring up to eight times a day, and lasting for 15 minutes to three hours at a time. Pains come in bouts (hence 'cluster') lasting several weeks with remission lasting months or years. This is one of the few types of headache where men are affected more often than women, the ratio being three to one. Ipsilateral autonomic disturbance is common, with facial sweating; and even Horner's syndrome (conjunctival injection, miosis and ptosis) may occur. Treatments are not very effective. *Lithium* is probably the best, and high dose steroids may abort a cluster. Ergot can help, pizotifen is not as good as methysergide, NSAIDs can help. Treatment with oxygen may relieve an acute attack within ten minutes.

Chronic paroxysmal hemicrania is different from cluster headache only in the brevity of the attacks, which last for minutes only (range three to 45 minutes). The pains invariably resolve completely with indomethacin, which may also be used in doses of 25 to 100 mg a day to prevent attacks.

Trigeminal neuralgia causes an intermittent burning pain which occurs in the distribution of the trigeminal nerve. Cold wind and eating typically aggravate the symptoms. Carbamazepine is the treatment of choice, followed by phenytoin.

Miscellaneous headaches

Those in this group are so obscure they don't even fit into one of the International Headache Society's 13 categories. Highlights include

- *Ice pick headache* or *cephalalgia fugax*. There are intense head pains which last a fraction of a second only. They often occur in migraine sufferers. Indomethacin is the treatment of choice
- *External compression headache* results if a cutaneous cephalic nerve is compressed, for instance by swimming goggles
- *Benign exertional headache* comes on with exercise, and is often like migraine in character. A worrying variant is associated with sexual activity. Propranolol and indomethacin often help
- *Coital cephalalgia, thunderclap headache* and *exploding head syndrome* all have an acute onset. Their first presentation will often require hospital admission
- *Cervical spondylosis* is very common in older people and may give rise to headaches.

A consultation for headache

Even though headaches are common, they can also indicate serious and life-threatening illness. Most people with headache do not consult a doctor about them. Those that do *must have their reasons*.

- The headaches may have become more severe or frequent
- The pattern of the headaches may have changed
- They may be interfering with some aspect of normal life
- The sufferer may have specific fears about the headache, perhaps prompted by a television programme or an acquaintance who has headaches caused by something serious
- There may be anxiety or depression present which is not only making the headaches worse, but also making the patient worry more about them.

A *full assessment* should be made *at least once* in all patients who choose to consult with headache. The rare instance of serious pathology must not be missed. Fears and concerns must be explored and discussed. Patients must feel that they have had a proper hearing and are being taken seriously. At some stage patients with tension headache will have to be told why they have their pain, and that available treatments are not very good: such a discussion can only go well if there is shared understanding and trust.

Questions to ask[24]

- *How long has the headache been present, and have you had similar headaches in the past?* A prolonged duration of identical symptoms precludes any progressive pathological process
- *Is the headache recurring or persistent?* Migraine is episodic and there is complete relief between attacks. Tension headache is more persistent
- *Where is the headache?* Cervical spine or neck muscle problems can cause pain arising from the neck and spreading upwards. Tension headaches are usually all over the head. Migraine is frequently one sided
- *How long does the headache last?* Migraines last a maximum of 72 hours
- *Are there any associated symptoms?* 25% of migraine sufferers get an aura. Neurological symptoms may be part of migraine, but the question of intracranial pathology should also be addressed
- *Are nausea and vomiting present?* 95% of migraine sufferers have nausea and/or vomiting (and 20% have *diarrhoea*). Tension headache may cause nausea but not vomiting. Effortless vomiting is associated with raised intracranial pressure
- *What makes the headache better?* Sleep, dark and quiet improve migraine attacks
- *What brings the headache on?*
- *What drugs are you taking?* This will be an assessment of the severity of the pain, its response to treatment and the possibility of analgesic headache. Tension headache responds poorly to analgesics
- *Do you have any specific worries about the headache?* Sometimes the headache will be disrupting work or a favourite hobby. There may be concern about a brain tumour, raised blood pressure or an imminent stroke. Making a specific enquiry about concerns is the best way of unearthing them.

Useful address

The Migraine Trust
45 Great Ormond Street
London WC1N 3HZ
Telephone: 020 7831 4818

Suggested examination

A clinical examination *rarely* reveals useful information. However it will be expected by the patient, and contributes to the sense that the problem is being taken seriously. An examination also has medico-legal importance as a missed serious diagnosis can have severe repercussions.

📄 **Guidelines**

Physical examination for headache[20]

- CNS examination including cranial nerves and fundi, but papilloedema is only found in around 50% of cases of brain tumour[21]
- Movements of the cervical spine and temporomandibular joints
- Gentle pressure to the sinuses, and also the temporal arteries in the over-50s
- Auscultate the carotid arteries
- Measure the blood pressure.

Except with very high levels raised blood pressure does not cause headache, but this is not common knowledge. Since most patients have this belief, they will be perplexed if the doctor does not measure their blood pressure, will be dissatisfied with their consultation and will probably not follow advice. Checking the BP ensures that a thorough assessment job has been done, and is also an opportunity for screening.

Referral

Reasons to refer to hospital a patient with headache include:

- Treatment not working
- Patient request
- Diagnostic doubt
- Medication misuse headache
- More than one type of headache
- Sinister features present.

📄 **Guidelines**

Sinister features of headache[11]

- Recent onset severe headache in patient over 50
- Progressive headache
- Morning headache, vomiting
- Neurological deficit or seizure
- Possible papilloedema
- Known malignancy or endocrine dysfunction.

Summary

- Nearly everyone gets a headache from time to time
- The commonest primary cause of headache is tension, the commonest secondary cause of headache is fever
- Only a minority of people with headache consult a doctor. A diagnosis of tension headache should be made positively, and not just by exclusion

- It is rare to start with migraine over age 40
- Brain tumours and other serious causes of headache are very rare, but must not be missed. Any suspicion of a serious diagnosis makes urgent referral mandatory
- Amitriptyline is the best available treatment for chronic tension headache, and may also help any associated depression. However it rarely completely cures the problem
- Patients with headache often have their lives made miserable. They deserve a sympathetic hearing and realistic management.

✎ Topics for discussion

- GPs should have open access to MRI/MNR scanners
- Patients should self-medicate for their headaches
- Tension headache and 'heart-sink patient' often go together
- Conventional medicine has little to offer for tension headache
- Patients tend to refer to any troublesome headache as migraine. Why?
- The best emergency treatment for acute migraine is intra-muscular opiate
- Migraine sufferers would do well to consult an alternative practitioner.

📖 References

1. Ritchie S A and Bates D. Primary and secondary headache. *Update* 1998; 56: 270.
2. Lane R J M. Is it migraine? The differential diagnosis. *Update* 1991; 43: 760.
3. Marshall J. Frequent headache often results in absence from work. *Medical Monitor* 11 November 1998: 46.
4. Goadsby P J and Olesen J. Diagnosis and management of migraine. *BMJ* 1996; 312: 1279–83.
5. Fowler T J. Management of headache. *Update* 1991; 43: 635–53.
6. Abu-Arefeh I and Russell G. Prevalence of headache and migraine in school children. *BMJ* 1994; 309: 765–9.
7. Fearon P and Hotopf M. Relation between headache in childhood and physical and psychiatric symptoms in adulthood: national birth cohort study. *BMJ* 2001; 322: 1145–8.
8. Migraine: costs and consequences. *Bandolier* 1999; 6(9): 5–6.
9. Fontebaso M. Set realistic goals for management of headache. *Medical Monitor* 13 January 1999: 42–3.
10. Peatfield R. How should GPs treat migraine? *Monitor* 1995; 8(17): 43–6.
11. Bullock P. Headache: Part 1. *General Practitioner* September 1 2000: 34–5.
12. Ostergaard J R. Warning leak in subarachnoid haemorrhage. *BMJ* 1990; 301; 190–1.
13. Mason J C and Walport M J. Giant cell arteritis. *BMJ* 1992; 305; 68–9.
14. Khunti K. Management of headache. *Update* 1997; 54: 557–9.
15. Management of tension-type headache. *Drug and Therapeutics Bulletin* 1999; 37(6): 41–4.
16. MacGregor E A. Prescribing for migraine. *Prescribers' Journal* 1993; 33(2): 50–8.
17. Clough C. Non-migrainous headaches. *BMJ* 1989; 299: 70–2.
18. 'Minerva'. *BMJ* 1996; 312: 1490.
19. Managing migraine. *Drug and Therapeutics Bulletin* 1998; 36(6): 41–4.
20. Hackett G. Management of migraine. *The Practitioner* 1994; 238: 130–6.

21. Kenny C. Headaches and migraines. *Horizons* 1992; 6: 430–3.

22. MacGregor A. Make sure the symptoms point clearly to migraine. *Horizons* 1993; 7: 390–4.

23. Chang C L, Donaghy M, Poulter N, and World Health Organisation. Collaborative Study of Cardiovascular Disease and Steroid Hormone Contraception. *BMJ* 1999; 318: 13–18.

24. Wilkinson M. Management of headache. *The Practitioner* 1992; 236; 449–51.

Loss and bereavement

Tutorial aim	**The registrar can plan a programme of support for a bereaved patient.**
Learning objectives	By the end of the tutorial the registrar can:

- List four stages of a normal grief reaction and describe each stage
- List four categories of 'at risk' bereaved people
- Discuss the appropriate use of medication in bereavement
- Identify abnormal grief
- Choose an agenda for contacts with the bereaved

>   at death
>   after the funeral
>   at four months

- List the requirements of a practice bereavement protocol
- Decide when further intervention is needed, and choose appropriate care.

A loss reaction

Bereavement is *being robbed of anything we value.*[1] However, the word usually implies that someone has died, and this meaning will be used in these notes. When someone suffers a loss which affects a number of different aspects of their life a typical reaction results: a *loss reaction*. As well as resulting from the death of someone close, a loss reaction can be produced by

- Amputation or other loss of body parts
- Blindness and other loss of sensory or cognitive functions
- Disabling illness
- Effects of ageing:

>   memory loss and dementia
>   loss of appetites, including sexual appetite
>   risk of serious disease and loss of assumption of health
>   reduced mobility
>   contemporary friends dying off

- Social loss: divorce, redundancy
- Children become bereaved if their parents divorce.

Grief is the psychological reaction to a bereavement, but reactions to any loss can follow the same pattern. Since recurrent loss is an inevitable part of the human condition, understanding the loss reaction is essential for all who would offer care and support. The significance of a loss can only be understood by the person who is undergoing it.[2] Understanding a loss requires knowledge of the sufferer's frame of reference, which may be not at all what you expect. The best way to find out what someone is thinking is to ask. Grief may begin when a fatal diagnosis is made: there is grief for lost health and loss of future life, and the family grieve in anticipation of their loss to come. Grief in anticipation of a death tends to become more intense as the death approaches, whereas following a death the grieving process generally becomes less troublesome with the passage of time.

Statistics of death

- The death rate in the United Kingdom is about 12 per 1000 people per year
- There are about 600 000 deaths each year, and 1.5 million people a year suffer a major bereavement[3] by death
- A GP with a list of 2000 patients can expect 25 deaths among patients each year. Of these 15 will be over 70 years and two will be under 45 years old. At any one time there will be up to two terminally ill patients
- Sixty per cent of people die in hospital.

▱ Evidence

Bereaved of spouse[4]	
Men aged 45 to 59	2%
Men over 75	30%
Women 45 to 59	8%
Women over 75	64%
Total UK population bereaved of spouse	4 million (135 per average GP list)

The GP's involvement in bereavement

The bereaved population will come to the GP's attention in a number of ways.

- **Mortality.** The chance of death following a bereavement is increased between 10[5] and 600%.[4] Increased mortality is greatest in the first six months for widowers and in the second year for widows. Men and the younger bereaved are at greater risk.[4] There is no particular illness which causes these excess deaths, but coronary heart disease and alcohol abuse are well represented. Suicide is also more common in the first year after a bereavement. In years past infectious diseases were particularly prevalent. Two hundred years ago the Registrar General allowed 'grief' as a legitimate cause of death on a death certificate.[6]
- **Morbidity.** Psychological illness is increased by bereavement. The use of alcohol and prescribed drugs often increases after bereavement. Physical morbidity may also be increased, but studies on this are inconclusive.[7]

📁 **Evidence**

Morbidity following bereavement	
One year after a bereavement[8] the bereaved may	
feel health 'not good'	50%
be admitted to hospital	30%
suffer major depression	12%

- The chance of clinical depression and anxiety among widows and widowers is about a quarter in the first year, falling to about a fifth by the end of the first year, and declining thereafter.[9]
- **Bureaucracy.** Every death has to be certified by a registered medical practitioner. The terms used on the death certificate may be confusing and need explaining to the bereaved family.
- **Continuity.** The GP will often have built up a relationship over many years with the deceased and their family. If the terminal care and death have been at home, then the relationship between GP and family will have been particularly intense. It is appropriate to continue this care at what is a distressing time.
- **Efficacy.** The involvement of a GP or other carer in a counselling role after a bereavement is possibly of some benefit[4], though conclusive evidence is lacking.[10]
- **GP's feelings.** Almost all GPs feel guilty about issues relating to the death of a patient.[10] This may be the result of close relations built up over years, or because the bulk of GP training is still done in hospitals where death is the ultimate medical failure. Some GPs are struggling with unresolved grief of their own.

The stages of grief

It is often possible to identify distinct stages in how a person reacts to a loss. The severity and length of the stages will vary from person to person, and some people may miss out a stage or stages altogether. Understanding that grief is a process within which *milestones* can be identified is helpful for the bereaved and their carers: the process has to be gone through, but each new phase means that progress toward eventual resolution is being made. A full grief reaction often takes over a year to complete, and a duration of up to two years is common. The following four stages are recognized.

1. Numbness

This can last for a few hours or up to a week. The reality of the death has not sunk in, as though the bereaved needs time to catch up with the present. Normal functioning is suspended, and help may be needed with purposeful thinking and action. The bereaved may deny or try to bargain away reality: 'perhaps a mistake has been made'; 'perhaps I will wake out of this nightmare'. This stage is characterised by free-floating *anxiety and sleeplessness*.

2. Pining

This tends to begin about the time of the funeral, and may last for a month or so. The funeral is a particularly important ritual which finally confirms the death so that it can no longer be wished away. The grieving person will often want to see and touch the body. If this contact is denied either because of circumstances or because a misguided well-wisher forbids it, then the progress of the grief may be blocked.[11] There may be overactivity of a *searching* nature. Cupboards may be cleared out obsessively, as though the deceased is being looked for.

Anger and guilt may be apparent. The bereaved may feel that the death is so unfair that someone must be to blame for it. If these feelings are turned inwards guilt results. It is not uncommon for anger to be directed at the GP or other doctors involved in the terminal illness. The GP should maintain a professional detachment in these circumstances, but if the anger is too great then that particular GP may have to withdraw from the case. Another feature of this stage is the need repeatedly to go over the events leading up to the death, often in meticulous detail. This can happen particularly when the bereaved has not been present at the death.[12] Offering the bereaved a chance to review the events leading up to the death is therapeutic. The doctor's role is to explain any medical details, and offer repeated assurance that neither the bereaved nor anybody else is to blame for the death.

3. Disorganisation and despair

When the funeral is over and the rest of the family have returned to their own homes, the consequences of the death begin to be realised, leading to *pangs of acute distress*. Distress may be brought on by a recollection, or an object: after years of marriage the house will be littered with memories. The distress may be so severe that bizarre behaviour arises, leading the bereaved to think they are going mad. There may be a strong sense of the *deceased's presence*, so that the bereaved may feel they have 'heard' the deceased's voice or more uncommonly have 'seen' the deceased, usually in a familiar setting. After years of marriage, couples can predict with some accuracy what their partner is going to do or say in particular circumstances. These memories are so strong that they creep into reality. Depression is a normal and healthy reaction to bereavement.

4. Reorganisation

The reality of the new world without the deceased is now apparent, and adjustments begin to be made to cope. This stage is the longest and can persist up to two years. Even after this time the deceased is not forgotten, but their absence is being tolerated. *'I will not insult you by telling you that one day you will forget. I know that you will not. But at least in time you will not remember as fiercely as you do now, and I pray that time may be soon.'*[13] Waves of distress may persist, and pining may recur, especially when *provoked by a memory or an event*. During the first year it is always possible to think back to what happened this time last year. Family occasions, birthdays, Christmas and anniversaries are poignant times. Meeting people who are unaware that the death has occurred causes distress to both parties. The resumption of normal social activities, or the first time the bereaved experiences enjoyment or laughs can trigger guilt feelings again. Many bereaved people find that the middle months of the first year after the death are particularly hard to endure.[3]

Predicting abnormal grief

Up to 30% of those who are bereaved will develop abnormal grief.[14] Even with a normal reaction, there may be evidence of significant distress in up to a quarter of the bereaved at two years.[15]

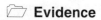 **Guidelines**

Predictors of abnormal grief:[9,16]

- Death of spouse
- Untimely death of young person
- Death of parent (particularly in early childhood and adolescence)
- Sudden death, especially if gruesome
- Multiple deaths, particularly disasters
- Stigmatised death: suicide, AIDS
- Deaths by murder or manslaughter
- Caring for deceased for over six months
- Unable to carry out valued religious rituals.

People at risk:
- Ambivalent relationship with deceased. The initial distress is less, but the guilt and sense of searching are more severe and prolonged (up to four years).
- Dependent relationship with deceased. When all aspects of the couple's life are intertwined, every event is a reminder of the loss. In addition, some essential skills of daily living which were previously the domain of the deceased may need to be relearned. For the widower whose wife did all the cooking, not only will he have to learn how to cook for himself, but each time he does so will be a reminder of his loss. A sense of *yearning and loneliness* persists.
- Low self-esteem
- Little trust in others
- Multiple previous bereavements
- Prior mental illness, especially depression
- Poor perceived social support
- Other life stresses.

Evidence

The Harvard study of abnormal bereavement[17]

A study of young widows 13 months after their bereavement showed a good outcome:

- After sudden death 9%
- After expected death 56%
- After a high conflict relationship with deceased 30%
- After a low conflict relationship with deceased 60%.

Detecting abnormal grief

No reaction

Grief may get 'stuck' so that it does not progress to the next stage. In some cases there may seem to be no reaction at all. There is evidence that the repression of emotions may be psychologically harmful.[18] The visible manifestations of grief have a strong social component. In Britain the openness of the Victorians about death was replaced with the 'stiff upper lip' mentality of the 1920s, possibly as a result of the national distress caused by deaths in the First World War.[18]

Men are less likely to express their grief than are women. In most Arab countries and in Africa death is accompanied by much wailing and public grieving. On the other hand, in Rwanda it is normal to show little grief. In cultures where bravery is revered, such as the Apache Indians, or in religions such as Buddhism where living is only a brief preparation for better things to come, there is little public display of grief.[18]

Help and treatment will be appropriate only if the person becomes ill because of their suppressed grief. People are rational, and will be stoical for their own good reasons. You may not understand those reasons, but that does not matter. If someone who is bereaved takes comfort from their behaviour, it should not be challenged. Suppressed grief is only a problem if it causes unwelcome symptoms.

Anger

Persisting anger may be a problem, and this can be made worse if an inquest has been needed or if a complaint has been registered about a doctor involved in the care of the deceased. In either of these events there may be a significant delay in all the facts surrounding the death being clarified. The activation of a complaints procedure nearly always means that the doctors/professionals concerned will try to defend their actions.

Pining

Prolonged pining or searching, morbid preoccupation with death, a history of psychiatric illness or persisting guilt all predict a poor outcome. The suggestion that the grief has not resolved often comes from a carer.

Depression

Depression is a normal feature of the early and middle phases of grief. This cannot be altered by treatment, and indeed antidepressants may make matters worse by delaying progression to the further stages of grief. However, treatable depression is also very common following bereavement, and it is often difficult to judge where normal depression finishes and clinical depression starts. The depression of grief can affect appetite, sleep patterns, motivation and the will to live. There should, however, be a trend for grief depression to improve with time, and by *six months* many of the symptoms should be abating.[9]

📄 Guidelines   Treating depression after bereavement[9]

Treatment should be considered for depression when:

- Symptoms are severe
- There are episodes of or danger of self-harm
- Depression continues more than six months after the death.

Sometimes a therapeutic trial with antidepressants can help to clarify the situation.

Prolonged grief

Some people never fully work through a grief reaction, and though in many respects they are functioning normally there are nonetheless signs of distress. Grief may be described with *freshness* even though the death was years before. Minor triggers provoke intense distress. Themes of loss keep appearing in discussion. The bereaved is unwilling to move the deceased's possessions, in what seems like an attempt to *deny* the loss. Physical symptoms like those of the deceased may develop. Radical lifestyle changes may be made.

Helping the bereaved

Bereavement is a natural and normal process and there is no cure for it. A good network of supportive relationships helps the bereavement progress normally. Professional and voluntary carers may supplement the patient's own social support network. Short-term *counselling* can be helpful in securing a normal grief reaction,[15] particularly counselling directed at those in 'high-risk' categories.[16] The best environment for the bereaved is one in which they can *express their feelings freely* and still be accepted. Confidants who have undergone a bereavement themselves are particularly helpful.

🖹 **Guidelines**

The role of carers in bereavement

- Understand and be available[1]
- Listen rather than talk
- Reinforce the normality of what is happening
- Accept that there will inevitably be displays of anger, guilt and distress
- Counsel against major life changes, especially in the early stages of a bereavement reaction. Some bereaved people want to make a clean break with the past. Some, possibly encouraged by well-wishers, want to uproot and move house: this is nearly always a mistake.

Hindering the bereaved

Many people find the distress of others distressing. It is a bit un-English to give way to displays of emotion. Carers may be upset by what is going on, and will say and do things which are probably unhelpful to the bereaved. The encouragement to the bereaved to suppress their emotions is reinforced by the rituals surrounding death. Cremation may be quick and hygienic, but there is little left for the bereaved to mourn. Death is not talked of, except in hushed tones, and is certainly not a subject for pleasant conversation. It is not considered appropriate to speak ill of the dead, so discussion is clouded by a lack of full openness and honesty.

📁 **Evidence**

> **Hindering grief[15]**
>
> Unhelpful attitudes identified by the bereaved include:
>
> - Offers of advice
> - Attempts to encourage recovery
> - Forced cheerfulness
> - False empathy, such as, 'I know how you feel . . .'

The use of medication

In the early days of a bereavement distress may be overwhelming, and sleep impossible. It is often appropriate to prescribe a small quantity of anxiolytic such as diazepam 5 mg three times a day to help over the first day or so. Lack of sleep may be an extra worry in that some people feel that this may lead to illness. Once assured on this point, night sedation is often declined.

Tablets will not cure bereavement, and by reducing awareness may actually impede the grief process. Most people will accept this, and it is not uncommon for only a few doses of the medication to be taken. Confronting the distress head on is hard work at the time, but probably means that the adjustment to the new reality of life without the deceased progresses more rapidly. Some people will reject any medication because they want to confront their grief head on. They will have their own reasons for doing this, and so the eventual outcome is likely to be better. Facing the intensity of grief head on may be preferred by the bereaved because:

- They may feel that this is the best and quickest way of achieving recovery. They are probably correct
- There may be a feeling that a supreme effort has to be made in recognition of the magnitude of the loss. At one level this can be seen as a part of a denial process where the bereaved seems to be trying to *overcome reality* by their efforts. At another level, hard work is widely regarded in our culture as an appropriate way of solving a problem, and it also provides a channel for any restless anxiety the bereaved may be feeling
- Some bereaved people are concerned that they are not grieving in the right way. For them only a public display of extreme distress is sufficient recognition of the loss; otherwise it might look as though they didn't really care. Bereaved people who feel some guilt regarding the death may be more prone to such a reaction.

The routine use of antidepressants does not help grief. However if major depression does occur it should be treated like any other depression using antidepressant medication in full doses.

The GP's role

Breaking bad news

The GP may be involved in telling the family that a death has occurred or is likely to occur. It is important to break the news in such a way that the message is got across without causing unnecessary distress. A more detailed discussion on how to break bad news can be found in the chapter on Terminal Care.

📄 Guidelines

Breaking bad news[19]

- Make protected time available
- Deliver information slowly to prevent denial. Pause between pieces of information
- Be honest without being brutally honest. Do not make promises which you are unable to fulfil
- Try to assess the immediate reaction and answer initial questions. Answers may be modified by the bereaved's reactions. Some people will require medical information in considerable detail, while others show little reaction and ask no questions
- Explore the bereaved's concerns and make time to deal with them. Reflecting the questions is a good way of exploring the bereaved's true feelings.

At Death

Attend promptly – This is not a medical emergency, but it is a social one. Little can be achieved in terms of counselling, but the bereaved will usually welcome a visit.[20] There are some practical issues which may need discussing such as undertakers, death certificates and registration of the death. Sometimes physical contact helps. If the death is expected, carers may feel confident enough to contact the undertaker directly, so that the GP's visit can be delayed to a more convenient time. Medication may be appropriate, as described in the previous section.

In the few weeks after a death, the bereaved will be deluged with requests for information. Pension and insurance companies will often need proof of death. There may be immediate financial concerns. Further information can be obtained from the undertaker, from the local social services department or from the DSS booklet *What to do after a death.*[21]

There is no formal mechanism by which a patient's GP is informed of a death. A minority of patients will be seen immediately after death by the GP or a partner. Information on the others may be more difficult to obtain. It is good practice for hospitals to ring a patient's GP at the earliest opportunity after a death in hospital. Other team members may become aware of a death. There may be a notice in the local press. However notification of a death is received, the information must be disseminated to any team member who may have dealings with the bereaved. Some practices keep a *Death Register,* entering patient details and also details of persons who may be affected by the loss. Any hospital departments should be notified. There is little more distressing for the bereaved and embarrassing for the GP than the receipt of an outpatient appointment after someone has died. The *date of the death* should be entered into the bereaved's medical records. This can be useful in future contacts.

After the funeral

In some cases it will be deemed appropriate to review the bereaved at the surgery. However, review at home is probably better[1] because

- The bereaved are in their own surroundings

- Time is not as limited as it might be with a surgery appointment system
- It saves the distress of waiting in the waiting room.

Though an early review of progress is useful, care should be taken so that the GP does not turn up on the day of the funeral, except in a personal capacity.

On the agenda for this review:

- The family have gone home and the house is empty. At around two weeks the bereaved will experience lots of guilt feelings and searching. They will want to go through the *details of the death*
- Explain anything on the death certificate which is not understood.
- Discuss the events leading to the death if the patient wishes
- Describe grief reactions and emphasise that they are normal. Feelings of anger and depression are normal, as is seeing and hearing the deceased
- Assess what support is available. This may be family, friends, clergymen or voluntary groups.

If there is good support there may be no need for further intervention unless and until the bereaved requests it. Many undertakers provide a bereavement service, as do many community nurse teams and the Macmillan service if they have been involved with the deceased before death. Self-help organisations such as Cruse or Compassionate Friends may be appropriate sources of support. Cruse has 200 branches in the country and, in 1993, 22 000 bereaved people were counselled and 5000 attended local social support groups.

Self-help groups

Cruse
Cruse House, 126 Sheen Road,
Richmond TW9 1UR
Counselling Tel: 020 8332 7227
Information Tel: 020 8940 4818
Or local group

Compassionate Friends
53 North Street
Bedminster
Bristol, BS3 1EN
Tel: 0117 966 5202
Or local group

Support from the *church* can be particularly helpful. Clergymen receive specific training in the support of the bereaved, and are probably the professional group in the best position to offer support, especially where the bereaved already has contact with the church. For all those who wish to offer support to the bereaved, a sensitivity to spiritual needs is appropriate.

Around four months

This contact is optional, and depends on assessments done at previous visits. A consultation at about four months is particularly appropriate for those who are poorly supported, or for whom there have been concerns about the development of an abnormal reaction. The initial grief is often starting to resolve. The progress of the grief should be assessed. At this stage it should be clear whether or not the grief is likely to be normal. If there seem to be problems, then further contacts may be organised either at home or at the surgery.

If abnormal grief seems to be occurring, then

- Increase the frequency of contact with the bereaved
- Be alert for symptoms of major depression
- Refer on to either a professional or lay colleague
- Advise contact with a self-help group if this has not already been done.

A practice protocol for bereavement

Much of what might be considered good practice in the management of bereavement concerns organisational issues. Many practices have developed a protocol to be used after a death. Points to be included are:

- A central register in the practice where all deaths are notified. This can be a book or a form designed for the job
- All team members must know how to enter a death on the register. Information about a death may come from a number of sources
- Once notified, there must be a method whereby the fact of the death is disseminated to the professional groups who need to know. Within the practice this might be the nurses or physiotherapists. Outside the practice any outpatient departments offering ongoing care to the deceased should be told
- One professional should be identified as taking responsibility for the monitoring of the bereavement process in each case. This is often but not always a GP, and may be the GP who knows the relatives rather than the GP who looked after the deceased.
- If a GP or another professional does not feel it appropriate to visit the bereaved, then alternative means of contacting the family should be considered. This might be by letter – it is a good idea to have a pre-prepared draft – or by telephone contact. Some GPs feel that a visit might be intrusive but such a visit is seldom so regarded by the bereaved. Many GPs find bereavement visits difficult, but this should not influence their decision about what sort of contact with the bereaved is most appropriate.

Bereaved children

The response of children to loss is in many ways similar to that of adults, but *modified by their own perceptions.*[22] Deaths of first degree relatives are rare, but loss through divorce causes reactions just as severe as death, and by some measures (e.g. incidence of enuresis) causes more problems.[2] Similar reactions can be seen after the loss of a pet, or even after moving house.

The loss of a parent in childhood is associated with an *increased chance of psychiatric disorders*, particularly depression, in adult life.[23]

- If under six months of age the baby has no concept that people continue to exist when they can't be seen, and so there is no separation anxiety
- Under two years children have no idea of the permanence of death
- From two to seven years children see the world only from their own viewpoint, and may feel responsible that the loss has occurred
- From seven to twelve years there is acceptance that death is not their fault
- Over 12 years abstract thinking is such that hypothetical situations can be speculated on.

Typically, the following stages are gone through

- *Protest.* Anger, crying, looking for the parent
- *Despair.* Depression, hope of reunion lost
- *Emotional detachment.* Recovery is apparent, but the capacity to form deep attachments is damaged.

An abnormal reaction in a bereaved child is suspected if there is prolonged depression, scholastic failure, social isolation of more than three months, inability to play, antisocial or aggressive behaviour, drug or alcohol abuse, delinquency, sexual acting out, prolonged somatic symptoms or thoughts of suicide or dying.[2]

Summary

- A GP with an average list size will have 25 patients die each year, and 135 patients who are bereaved
- Bereavement carries a morbidity and a mortality. A GP will also be involved in the bureaucracy of death
- Nearly all GPs feel some guilt when one of their patients dies
- Bereavement cannot be cured by pills or anything else. Depression and distress, powerful emotions, are normal components of grief
- Normal grief can last two years or more. The dead person is not forgotten, but their absence is tolerated
- GP support for the bereaved is nearly always welcomed, and may be helpful
- Abnormal grief can to some extent be predicted from the circumstances of the death and factors in the life and personality of the bereaved
- Some of the bereaved will benefit from specialised bereavement counselling.

Topics for discussion

- The medicalisation of grief is an unforgivable intrusion into what is a normal human reaction
- The better the relationship, the more you miss it
- Grief can be avoided if you keep busy and try to forget what has happened
- Only doctors who have been bereaved themselves can be any good at working with the bereaved
- Which primary healthcare team member is best equipped to run the practice bereavement protocol? Should the choice be based on training or on personal characteristics?

📖 **References**

1. Charlton R and Dolman E. Bereavement: a protocol for primary care. *Br J Gen Pract* 1995; 45: 427–30.
2. Furnivall J and Wilson P. Coping with loss in childhood. *Medical Monitor* 1991; 4: 51–4.
3. Wallbank S. Cruse. *Well Woman* 1995; 18: 13–14.
4. McAvoy B R. Death after bereavement. *BMJ* 1986; 239: 835.
5. Martikainen P and Valkonen T. Mortality after death of a spouse in relation to duration of bereavement in Finland. *J Epidemiol Community Health* 1996; 50: 264–8.
6. Parkes C M. Recent bereavement as a cause of mental illness. *Br J Psychiatry* 1964; 110: 198–204.
7. Woof W R and Carter Y H. The grieving adult and the general practitioner: a literature review in two parts (part 1). *Br J Gen Pract* 1997; 47: 443–8.
8. Wilkes E. The dying patient; the medical management of incurable and terminal illness. Lancaster: MTP Press,1982.
9. Murray Parkes C. *Coping with loss* Bereavement in adult life. *BMJ* 1998; 316: 856–9.
10. Saunderson E M and Ridsdale L. General practitioners' beliefs and attitudes about how to respond to death and bereavement: qualitative study. *BMJ* 1999; 319: 293–6.
11. Cathcart F. Seeing the body after death. *BMJ* 1988; 297: 997–8.
12. Freeman R. Supporting the grieving patient. *Medical Monitor* 1991; 4: 33–4.
13. Rattigan T. Collected works. London: Hamilton, 1953.
14. Yates D W, Ellison G and McGuiness S. Care of the suddenly bereaved. *BMJ* 1990; 301: 29–31.
15. Preston J. The consequences of bereavement. *The Practitioner* 1989; 233: 137–9.
16. Sheldon F. *ABC of palliative care* Bereavement. *BMJ* 1998; 316: 456–8.
17. Parkes C M, Weiss R S. Recovery from bereavement. New York: Basic Books, 1983.
18. Murray Parkes C. Understanding grief across cultures. *Psychiatry in Practice* 1998; 17(4): 5–8.
19. McLaughlan C A J. Handling distressed relatives and breaking bad news. *BMJ* 1990; 301: 1145–9.
20. Main J. Improving management of bereavement in general practice based on a survey of recently bereaved subjects in a single general practice. *Br J Gen Pract* 2000; 50: 863–6.
21. What to do after a death. DSS leaflet No. D49. London HMSO.
22. Furnivall J and Wilson P. Coping with loss in childhood. *Medical Monitor* 1991; 4: 56–62.
23. Parkes C M and Birtchnell J. Bereavement. *Proc R Soc Med* 1971; 64: 279–82.

Managing your money in the early practice years

Tutorial aim	**The registrar can make adequate financial plans when entering general practice.**

Learning objectives	By the end of the tutorial the registrar can:
	
	• Describe how GP pay is determined
	• Detail expenses which can be claimed against tax
	• Describe how to keep records for tax purposes
	• List the main benefits of the NHSPS
	• Recall ways of augmenting pension
	• Plan for:
	
	    life insurance
	    locum insurance
	    ill-health insurance.

Background

The majority of general practitioners in Britain are *self employed*. Historically GPs have protected their self-employed status with much vigour. The argument is that it keeps the GP independent of the state and so able to deliver personalised care to patients unfettered by outside interference. There are also considerable tax advantages enjoyed by the self-employed.

The Doctors' and Dentists' Review Body (DDRB, or just *Review Body*) was set up in 1971 charged with advising the prime minister on the remuneration of doctors and dentists working in the NHS. In 1996 it was composed of eight people with backgrounds in administration and industry, *none of whom had current professional experience of the health service.*[1] From April 2001 the chair passed to barrister Michael Blair QC (no relation to the prime minister) who was previously counsel for the Financial Services Authority.[2] Each year, after taking evidence from the interested parties, the DDRB produces a report which the prime minister receives in January with a view to implementation in the following April.

The Review Body has the broad support of government and of the medical and dental professions as it offers the chance of avoiding direct confrontation between doctors and government. Any unresolved conflict could escalate into action (such as strike or work to rule) which might adversely affect patient care. Neither side wants this to happen. In order for the system to work properly the Review Body has to be truly independent, and government, the ultimate paymaster, has to abide by its recommendations. In 1993, for the first time, the Review Body refused to produce a report as the government had already announced that there was to be a pay ceiling in the whole public sector.

In its annual report the Review Body recommends levels of gross and net income for GPs, and then the levels of individual fees and allowances are juggled to try to achieve the required result. This means that not only is the average take-home pay of GPs calculated, but there is also a figure given for expenses. The figures for the year from April 2001 were £80 300 gross and £56 510 net of expenses for an average list size in England of 1846.[3] This takes account of average expenses of £23 790 which was actually a reduction from £24 510 the previous year. The figure of take-home pay of £56 510 masks a wide variation between GPs:

- Some practices will be more efficient than others in claiming all their item-of-service entitlements
- A number of GPs only do the minimum 26 hours at the practice. They are deemed to be 'full time' by the HA, but will not be drawing a full parity share of practice profits. This also distorts figures about the average GP list size
- Non-NHS income is not included. Practices with significant private work can boost their income considerably.

All this means that the average full-time GP will earn more than £56 510. In fact, the genuinely full-time GP in England can expect at parity around £73 000 a year.[4] The only way you can work out how much you might get in a particular practice is to look at the accounts and try to guess what the future might bring.

In addition there are an increasing number of general practice jobs coming available under the provisions of the *NHS (Primary Care) Act 1997*. These are based on locally agreed contracts, and many offer a salaried option for practitioners. They are proving particularly popular with recently trained GPs who seem in general more interested in the clinical work of general practice than the organisational and financial work. Most of the following notes apply to self-employed practitioners. Salaried GPs will be working under a different set of rules: for instance, the tax regulations are different, and the material on buying in to a practice may not be relevant.

Tax

When you join a partnership you are inextricably financially bound to your partners. Any lapse or error can be expensive and may cause a partnership dispute. Until April 1996 partnerships were collectively and severally liable for debts, including tax debts. This led to the occasional instance of outgoing partners refusing to pay their tax bills. If the partnership wished to continue in existence the remaining partners had to pay up. All that changed in 1996 when people in a partnership became individually liable for their tax debts, and tax became due on earnings in the current year rather than on those of the previous year.

Claims against tax

One of the benefits of being self employed (*schedule D tax*) is that work expenses are eligible for relief if they are *wholly and exclusively* incurred by the job. For the salaried employee on PAYE (schedule E tax), expenses are only allowed if they are wholly, exclusively and necessarily incurred. That one word *necessarily* can make a huge difference, and is very much subject to how the Inland Revenue defines it.

Allowable expenses are added on to the part of income which is deducted before the tax liability is assessed. Effectively this means that the tax relief is allowed at the top tax rate paid. For most GPs this is at present 40%. Expenses may quite properly be claimed against tax for the items listed below. Salaried GPs may also be able to make a claim, but convincing the Inland Revenue of the eligibility of the claim may be more difficult because schedule E rules apply. Some salaried posts offer augmented pay to compensate for this tax disadvantage.

- *Motoring.* This includes petrol, repairs and servicing, road fund licence, insurance, breakdown organisation membership, car rental costs, parking costs and any other expenditure arising because of motoring (but not fines imposed through parking or motoring offences). Relief is also available on loans taken out to buy vehicles, and on the depreciation of vehicles of 25% per year subject to a maximum of £3000 a year.[5] When you sell a car, however, the actual amount you sell it for is taken account of for tax purposes. It is usual to make claims for two cars in case of breakdown
- *Staff and clerical.* This will include salaries of employed reception and nursing staff etc., as well as recruiting, training and advertising costs. It is also legitimate to pay your spouse for practice work, such as on-call telephone answering and clerical assistance. This is most beneficial if the spouse is not otherwise working, but it may still be worthwhile if the spouse is paying a lower rate of tax than the GP. The Inland Revenue has recently become interested in GPs who pay their spouse, and in many instances have challenged the legitimacy of the amount paid. If your accountants have experience of GP work they should be able to give an idea of what pay level is reasonable
- *Telephone charges*, both practice and domestic
- *Subscriptions, Journals, Postage, Stationery*
- *Drugs and requisites*
- *Household costs.* When the GP's private dwelling is used for consultations from time to time, it is not hard to convince the Inland Revenue of the legitimacy of a claim for household expenses. In other cases, a small amount may be claimed for other practice work done at home, or for equipment used for work purposes but kept at home. If dangerous drugs

are stored it is allowable to claim for the installation and servicing costs of a burglar alarm

- *Bank charges*. Accountancy and legal costs
- *Clothes cleaning*. It is assumed that a GP will wish to maintain a clean and tidy appearance
- *Pension plans and superannuation*
- *Study courses and other expenses*
- *Repairs and renewals*. You cannot claim tax relief on a new piece of equipment unless it is a replacement for an existing piece of equipment. Don't invest in the most expensive stethoscope and ophthalmoscope when you are a registrar, but wait till you are on schedule D and then replace the equipment with something decent
- *Locum insurance premiums*. It is a good idea to get insurance against any locum costs incurred if you are off sick. Premiums are allowed against tax, but any benefits are taxable. It is also possible to take out *permanent health insurance*, insuring your income against being permanently unable to work. Premiums on permanent health insurance policies are not tax allowable, but on the other hand any benefits are not taxed
- *Other practice expenses*. Professional indemnity insurance (defence society membership) is a significant professional expense. Even if it is paid through the practice, it should appear as a personal expense in your own accounts.

Keeping records for tax

Practice and work expenses fall into four broad categories:

1. Some practice expenses such as rent, rates, staff costs, locum charges etc. are best monitored by the practice administrative team. Expenses generated in this way are shared round the partnership.
2. Other individually incurred expenses may be paid for by the practice and so appear in the main practice accounts. Practices vary in this respect, so in some cases defence society membership and motoring expenses may be paid by the practice, while in others they fall to the individual doctor.
3. The third category of expenses comprises those which are paid partly by the practice and partly by the doctor. This might include stationery costs, etc.
4. Other expenses are entirely the province of the individual doctor, and will include subscriptions, etc.

For the convenience of the practice and the Inland Revenue, a number of *allowances* may be agreed in advance. This saves the GP having to produce proof of the expenditure and saves the Inland Revenue having to investigate. The Inland Revenue is allowed to scrutinise accounts for the *past six years* in cases of suspected minor fraud, and for *twenty years* for major fraud. Practices which have been subjected to an Inland Revenue investigation will confirm that it is expensive, laborious and time-consuming, and *to be avoided wherever possible*.

Any agreed allowances have to be *broadly reasonable* and not substantially out of step with other practices. Sometimes an agreed allowance is supplemented by a claimed amount. An example might be a practice allowance amount for stationery, with a further claim being made by the individual GP for proven extra expenditure.

In other cases it will be possible to claim for a proportion of the expenditure on a particular item. Typical of this type of agreement is the situation where a proportion of motoring costs are allowed so that you do not have to keep a car just for practice use. If the practice is not keeping a record of expenditure which it may be possible to claim against tax, then do so yourself. Records kept should be:

- In a book to form a permanent record
- Recorded at least monthly
- Supported where possible by vouchers (i.e. receipts).

Motoring expenses are often the most difficult to keep a track of. It is useful to keep a *credit card* to be used only for motoring expenses. The monthly accounts are adequate proof that the expenditure has been incurred.

Pensions

The NHS Pension Scheme (NHSPS)

A young GP just starting out in partnership will have many demands on the income. There may be the costs of a house move with a larger mortgage, perhaps a young child and a spouse unable to work. A new car may be needed. In addition there is the cost of buying in to the practice, and the professional indemnity insurance premium comes as a bit of a shock. Income is below parity (sometimes as low as half share at first) and expenses have not been accumulated to offset against tax. With all this going on a pension may be the last thing on your mind. Nonetheless it is important to give the subject a little thought for three reasons:

- This is the cheapest time to buy *added years*
- It is more expensive to top up your pension by any method when you are older
- You may be approached by an insurance company with a proposal to leave the NHSPS and join a commercial pension scheme.

The NHSPS costs you 6% of your superannuable income, which after tax relief is about 3% of your NHS income. In addition the health authority (HA) pays a further 4%. This money accumulates to form a *notional pension fund* which pays out on retirement. The benefits of the NHSPS will vary with individual circumstances. It pays an annual pension on retirement, plus a lump sum. Maximum benefits are payable after 40 years' service by age 60, or 45 years' service at age 65. The pension is *index linked* to the retail price index, and since the scheme is indemnified by the government it is as secure as you can get. Other benefits include:

- If you die, there is a pension for any surviving spouse and school age dependants

- Death gratuity if you die while still in post
- Partial and total disability benefits
- The British Medical Association will continue to negotiate improvements in the scheme even though you may have retired and left the practice.

Booklet SDP gives a guide to the major details of the NHSPS, and further advice can be obtained from either the pensions officer at the local HA, or direct from:

NHS Pension Scheme,
Hesketh House,
200–220 Broadway,
FLEETWOOD,
Lancashire FY7 8LG.
Tel: 01253 774910 (direct line)
        01253 774774 (switchboard)
        01253 774984 (fax)

Working out your pension entitlement

In practice this is very difficult. If you apply to the Fleetwood office they will give you an estimate, but this can only be relied upon in the year or so immediately before retirement. Superannuable income is not the same as actual income for two reasons:

- Private earnings are not included
- Some parts of income are assumed to be a reimbursement of expenses, and these are not superannuable.

This second factor makes pension entitlement particularly tricky to work out. Some payments from the HA are fully superannuable, while others are deemed to be solely reimbursed expenses. Of the rest, the partly pensionable, the current figure is that *66% are deemed superannuable*.[3] Your take-home pay is anyway net of practice expenses.

However, what you need to know is the amount of pension you are going to get. The easiest way of getting at this figure is to work it all out from the superannuation you pay in a year (figure available from the HA quarterly returns or the practice accounts), as this is 6% of your superannuable earnings.

The contributions which you and the HA make are paid into a personal pension fund. The retirement *pension is 1.4% of this fund per year*. You also get a *lump sum of 4.2% of the fund*. Clearly inflation has meant that money earned years ago is not as valuable now in purchasing terms. This is got round by the use of *dynamising factors*. These are set each year, and are figures by which actual money earned in a past year is multiplied to compensate for inflation. The dynamised amount is then added to the pension fund.

It is at present not clear what the pension arrangements will be for GPs who take a salaried option under the Primary Care Act.[6] The pension may well be rather less generous than that available to self-employed GPs. This is an important point for GPs seeking a salaried contract to clarify with their employer.

Working out how much pension you need

This will depend on your plans and priorities, and so no one can tell you. It will probably become a lot clearer as you get older, and this is also the time when you may have some spare money to do something about it. The sort of questions worth asking yourself are:

- Will the house be paid for?
- Will the children be independent?
- By how much will professional expenses fall?
- What will motoring and holiday requirements be?
- Do I intend to have a significant estate to leave?
- Will I want to move house?
- How long am I likely to live?

Other pensions

All reputable independent advisers suggest that GPs stay in the NHSPS since it is such a good scheme. A commercial pension offering the same level of benefits, in particular the index linkage, would be very expensive. In addition, on leaving the NHSPS you forego the HA contribution to your pension fund.

Up to a limit tax relief can be claimed on money paid into a pension fund. At age 35 the limit is 17.5% of income, and this rises in stages so that 40% of income paid into a pension at age 61 is allowable against tax.[3]

The A9 concession

The A9 concession is allowed by the Inland Revenue only for GPs and dentists. Under this you can opt to forego all tax relief on NHSPS contributions, and instead claim relief on premiums paid into another scheme. The percentage of income which can be paid into the pension fund is increased because you can pay in monies up to the limit for your age (you are not restricted to 6% of superannuable income plus any added years). The income on which the tax-allowable pension premiums is assessed is also increased because

- All income, not just superannuable income, is assessed
- Private income is also included.

To benefit from the A9 concession you have to want and be able to pay more into an independent scheme than you pay to the NHSPS. This really only makes sense if you have a lot of spare cash which you want to invest in a tax-efficient way.

Topping up the pension

There are broadly two options to top up the pension: to buy added years from the NHSPS or to buy a pension on the commercial market.

Added years

Many GPs will want to retire before they have completed the full 40 years' service which provides a maximum pension. It is now possible for GPs to retire at any age after 50 (or earlier if retirement is on the grounds of ill health), but the pension you get is correspondingly smaller: for instance at age 50 the pension is about 60% and the lump sum about 75% of what can be expected at age 60.[3] The shortfall can be got over to a degree by buying *added years* of pension benefit. You approach the NHSPS and apply to buy the added years. With their agreement extra contributions to the scheme are subtracted from income before the HA pays you. The HA makes no contribution to added-years agreements. The earlier you start buying added years, the cheaper it is. Exact details of how much it will cost can be obtained through the HA pension officer.

Additional voluntary contributions (AVCs)

There are other ways of topping up pension through the private sector, and buying added years is not particularly cheap. Some GPs will find the security of a government scheme more compelling than relying on the ups and downs of the stock market. On the other hand you can only back out of an added-years agreement under exceptional circumstances. Private sector schemes will accept variable payments at variable times, and so are much *more flexible*.

If you wish to top up your pension with a private scheme, this can be done either by approaching an insurance company of your choice or by getting a financial adviser to arrange it for you. Fees and commission paid to brokers for setting up these schemes can amount to up to half of the premiums paid in the first few years. The NHSPS has negotiated special terms with the *Equitable Life Insurance Society*, and so schemes arranged through them should be cheaper: it is not yet clear how this will be affected by Equitable Life's recent financial problems. AVCs will provide a pension, but not a retirement lump-sum.

In the early years in practice there are many pressures on the income and it is probably not necessary to get too much into debt in order to build up the pension at this stage. Bear in mind when planning any extra provision that there will almost certainly be extra assets in the form of lump sums available on retirement which can be used to top up the pension:

- The lump sum from the NHSPS
- Any share of practice assets.

The *cost-rent scheme* is a highly advantageous way of borrowing money for practice premises. A GP who owns a full share of their practice premises will have an asset of the order of £100 000. The cost-rent scheme allows the purchase of this asset with what is essentially an interest-free loan. This will contribute substantially to pension provision.

Insurance

The NHSPS provides a small amount of life insurance cover, but this is not much in the early years of service.

- *Term life assurance* can be taken out reasonably cheaply when you are young and fit. The cover should be enough to pay off your debts and give the family some security. Bear in mind that whatever level of cover you secure now, it will seem a lot less in 20 years' time
- Any loans taken out for substantial purchases (house, surgery) will usually require some sort of life cover assigned to them. An *endowment policy* is

only a with-profits life assurance, and so provides life cover as well as paying off the loan on maturity. In these days of low inflation, endowment policies have rather gone out of favour since they sometimes fail to mature to produce the required sum. However, unlike in house purchase, using an endowment to buy in to a practice is still tax-efficient as tax relief is allowable on interest at the maximum tax rate paid.

Dying is relatively easy in insurance terms. Inability to work because of temporary or permanent ill health is more difficult especially as the cost of living, if you are disabled, will probably go up.

The partnership agreement should contain details of what happens within the practice if a partner is unable to work because of *ill health*. It is usual, for instance, for a partnership to agree to provide cover for the first month of any sickness absence. The practice agreement should be read in conjunction with the *Statement of Fees and Allowances* (the Red Book) as, depending on the partnership list size, time in post of the sick doctor and the duration of absence, the practice may be eligible for *locum allowance* from the HA. It is usual for a practice agreement to require that the absent partner is responsible for meeting any locum costs incurred after the first month. On the other hand the absent partner receives any locum allowance available. The locum allowance is insufficient to meet the BMA recommended rates for a locum, so the amount has to be topped up. Locum allowance is only paid if a locum has been employed. After five years' NHS service a GP is entitled to locum allowance at full rate for six months and at half rate for a further six months. The key times in this scenario are after a month (when a locum is employed), after six months (when the locum allowance diminishes), and after a year (when the locum allowance stops). A number of insurance companies provide locum insurance policies to top up locum costs where benefits are deferred for the right length of time.

After a year's absence it is not unusual for the practice agreement to stipulate that the partnership dissolves and your income with it. It is possible to insure against this by taking out *permanent ill-health insurance*. The cost of premiums varies according to the size of benefit, and none of the ill-health policies will pay out more than 75% of final earnings in benefit. Index-linked benefits are best.

Locum insurance and income protection insurance are *getting more expensive* as more GPs retire early on the grounds of ill health. The best policies are those where the premiums and benefits are both index linked, but these are now not easy to find.

The insurance needs of the salaried GP will depend on the specific provisions of the contract agreed. Independent financial advice is probably a good idea.

Buying in

All practices need some working capital, and have some practice assets such as drugs and equipment. But by far the most costly practice asset is the surgery building if this is owned by the partnership. Any outgoing partner will want his or her share of practice assets, and this is normally paid for by the incoming partner.

It is always a good idea to check the buying-in procedure before accepting a partnership. The details should be in the partnership deed. Raising a large lump sum on relatively low earnings when there are other sizeable expenses can be difficult. If the capital involved is small, some practices allow the new partner an interest-free loan paid off over three to five years. With larger amounts buying in may be deferred until parity is reached. The method in closest accord with the legislation governing partnerships is for the incoming partner to be responsible for a share of capital proportional to profit share. If you start on a half parity share of profits, then you are responsible for half of the capital share of a full-parity partner.

Many young doctors will want to buy their share of the capital assets of the practice as a retirement fund, especially as by using the cost-rent scheme the purchase can be made at such favourable rates.

Some lenders may be prepared to allow you not to pay off the loan capital, so long as they continue to get their interest payments. The assets will remain with the partnership after you leave, and the debt will remain a partnership rather than a personal debt. If you wish to pay off the capital the options available are broadly similar to those available for house purchase, with the difference that tax relief at the highest rate paid is available on the interest for the whole loan.

While you are liable for a full share of the loan, you are also eligible for a full share of any cost-rent or notional-rent reimbursement from the HA. It is not unusual for all the interest to be covered by reimbursements, so that the only outlay for the GP is to pay off the capital.

Salaried GPs will usually not be involved in the capital of the practice, either buildings or goods and chattels.

Financial priorities

- If applicable, make sure that the Inland Revenue is aware that you wish self-employed tax status
- Make sure you are on any lists for which you are eligible, e.g. obstetric list, child health surveillance list
- Have a good close look at the accounts, and show them to your accountant. This should be done before signing the practice deed
- Think what would happen if you died in the near future
- Think what would happen if you were unable to work through ill health in the near future
- Make an initial appraisal of your pension provision. Check you are a member of the NHSPS. Consider added years. Other investments in pensions can be left till later when you might have some spare money.

Summary

- There are considerable financial benefits in being self employed. However, many young GPs prefer to be salaried under the provisions of the NHS (Primary Care) Act 1997

- The practice deed (agreement) should contain full details of how practice profits are to be allocated
- The cost of buying in to a practice is significantly offset by the benefits of the cost-rent scheme
- Exemption from tax can be claimed on a wide range of professional expenses. Proof of expenditure should be recorded at least monthly, in a bound book, and supported by receipts
- The NHS pension scheme is one of the best around
- No one can tell you how much pension you are going to need
- Life insurance is cheaper when you are younger
- For insurance purposes, death is much simpler than permanent disability
- Take independent financial advice sooner rather than later. Informal advice is usually readily forthcoming from senior GPs.

🗩 Topics for discussion

- Self-employed status for GPs encourages better patient care
- Good general practice is incompatible with maximising GP income
- Tax avoidance is as repugnant as tax evasion
- A good accountant will turn a blind eye to dubious expenses claims
- Salaried GPs are besmirching the proud traditions of British general practice.

📖 References

1. Anon. Altered Review Body Criticised. *General Practitioner* May 24 1996: 2.
2. BMA News 14 April 2001.
3. Database. *Medeconomics* 2001; 22(5): 67.
4. Anon. GP earnings up 10 per cent. *Best Practice* 6 June 2001: 7.
5. Budget taxation guide 1999. Sheffield: Barber, Harrison and Platt, Chartered Accountants, 1999.
6. An introduction to personal medical services. GPC, NAPC, NHS Alliance: London, 2000.

Referral to hospital

Tutorial aim	**The registrar can refer patients to hospital appropriately.**
Learning objectives	By the end of the tutorial the registrar can:

- List five reasons to refer a patient to hospital
- Describe three differences between specialist and GP decision-making methodologies
- List five requirements of a GP referral letter
- Discuss the advantages and disadvantages of the NHS referral system
- Describe one method of improving referrals
- Discuss with a patient an inappropriate referral request.

Statistics

The majority of general practitioners (GPs) refer to hospital between 23 and 41 cases per 1000 consultations.[1] However, there is a *large range* among all GPs from under 10 to over 170 referrals per 1000 consultations, a ratio of 23:1 between the highest and lowest referrers.[2] There is a fourfold difference in the referral rate between those GPs in the top fifth and those in the bottom fifth.[3]

In 1997/98 in the United Kingdom there were 41.6 million *outpatient* consultations.[4] About 11 million were new referrals, and 9 million of these were referred by GPs,[5] the rest having been internally referred within the hospital or from accident and emergency (A&E) departments.[6]

A parliamentary answer in 1997 estimated the average *cost* to the NHS of an outpatient attendance at £61[7] (£74.54 in 2001[8]). In addition it has been calculated that it costs each patient attending a hospital about £15 for a medical outpatient clinic and £23 for an attendance at an A&E department (2000).[9] The average cost of a general practice consultation is about £18, to which about £5 of patient cost should be added (2000).[9]

New outpatient referrals increased by 53% between 1949 and 1991.[10] During this time the number of GPs rose by 26%: the number of referrals per GP rose by 22%. This rise must be regarded as modest because an ageing population increases the need for treatment, and medical advances mean that more treatments exist for more conditions. Over the same period of time, the number of whole-time-equivalent consultants rose by 316%, and of junior hospital doctors by 253%: the average number of outpatients seen per consultant fell by 73% from 1680 to 618 a year.[10]

The ratio of *follow-up* to new outpatients, between 3 and 3.4 to 1, has remained remarkably steady. This however masks a wide variation in practice between different consultants. For instance, between surgeons there may be a fivefold difference in the number of follow-up appointments made after the same operation, without any obvious patient benefit.[11] Such figures have clear budgetary and contracting implications.

Between 5 and 38% of patients *fail to attend* their outpatient appointment, the commonest reasons being that they either forgot, or else due to a clerical error they were not informed of the appointment.[12]

Attendance at A&E departments has stayed remarkably steady at around 13.6 million a year.[4]

The history of the referral system

For many years the physicians held the upper hand among doctors in Britain. Their status was confirmed when the College of Physicians received royal patronage as early as 1518. Surgery on the other hand was performed by people with no medical qualifications. The status of surgery rose as the skill of surgeons improved, largely prompted by the activities of military surgeons. By 1800, when the Royal College of Surgeons of London was founded, surgeons considered their skills equal to those of physicians and both these groups were vying for control of the expanding number of hospitals.

Only the rich could afford the services of a physician or surgeon, and while these groups were fighting each other the poor turned to apothecaries for their healthcare. Some apothecaries were members of the Royal College of Surgeons, and some held a licentiateship of the Society of Apothecaries. Since the apothecaries were now caring for most of the population, it was inevitable that they should seek access to the hospitals, an access which would challenge the supremacy of the physicians and surgeons.

The Medical Acts of 1815 and 1858 were designed to resolve this dispute, as well as to ensure the adequacy of medical training (in 1858 there were 18 different institutions recognised by the General Medical Council for the issue of medical qualifications). A compromise was achieved: the physicians and surgeons would do mainly private work, but have unpaid 'honorary' appointments in the hospitals. The apothecaries were kept out of the hospitals, but their reward was that they became the only route through which the specialists could be consulted. 'The physicians and surgeons kept the hospitals, but the apothecaries kept the patients.'[13]

In the early nineteenth century, apothecaries began to call themselves general practitioners. The name was not universally liked: in 1830 a letter written to the *Lancet* commented that: '. . . *A more clumsy, more vulgar, or a more inapplicable expression could not have been found*'.[14]

By 1838, GPs were legally allowed to charge for their advice (previously they could only charge for medicines), and on 7 May 1845 a Bill was presented to parliament for the formation of a Royal College of General Practice. The Bill was not passed, and it was not until 19 November 1952 that the RCGP came into being.

Does the referral system work?

The National Health Service achieves morbidity and mortality rates broadly similar to those in the United States of America at about a third of the cost per person,[15] and broadly similar to France with half the number of doctors per head of population.[16] Even though there is significant variation in the availability of healthcare procedures and treatments within the NHS ('post-code rationing'), the variation in other countries between best and worst healthcare is much greater.

Why does the referral system work?

Though born of inter-professional rivalry the referral system has a compelling medical and political logic.

- About 90% of illness episodes which are presented to a doctor are treated by the GP only[17]
- The GP retains a *complete record* of all medical contacts
- The process of referral means that *two different medical opinions* with complementary views are involved in the personal and technical care of each patient.

Appropriate care

The care offered by GPs is different from the care offered by specialists. General practice is not an inferior version of hospital practice, it is a *separate specialty*.

A number of clinical conditions are never encountered in hospital because GPs deal with them: patients sent to hospital with these *GP conditions* are likely to receive sub-optimal and more expensive care.[18] For GP conditions, GPs are the appropriate specialists.

GPs patrol the margin between the NHS and the real world. Their key role is as the *interpreter of the interface between illness and disease*;[17] they sort out what the patient presents into a form which can be acted upon. There is more emphasis given to consultation skills in general practice education – both in vocational training and in continuing medical education – than in probably any other medical specialty.

The problem-solving *methodology* used by GPs, and their use of diagnosis based on that well-worn triad of physical, psychological and social factors, allows them to take a broad general view of patients' health needs. Patients who might benefit from specialist care can be identified, and referred on to the appropriate consultant. A referral to the wrong specialist will lead to unnecessary investigation and consequent lack of progress, plus extra tertiary (i.e. between consultant) referrals. A consultant is much more likely to seek the advice of another consultant when a problem outside their own specialty is identified even if the appropriate doctor for that problem is the patient's GP.

Sending a patient to the wrong consultant may end up being worse for the patient than if they had not been referred at all.

Clinical method

Most illness is not presented to a doctor at all, but is dealt with by the sufferer following discussion with family and friends. Symptoms are either endured or treated with something from the home medicine chest. Only about one in ten of all symptoms is presented to a doctor.[19] Much work has been done trying to work out why some patients choose to seek medical advice and others do not. The severity of the symptoms is only one of many factors which influence the decision.[20] In general it can be assumed that people with more severe symptoms are more likely to seek medical attention, but there is considerable overlap in symptom severity between the group who present and the group who do not.

Each GP will be well used to consulting with patients with a wide range of illnesses and symptoms. In most instances the illness can be left alone to recover by itself, or treated fairly simply. In deciding whether to refer a case, the GP's job is to identify patients who are *likely to benefit from specialist care*. Seeing the full range of symptoms and illnesses helps: of all doctors the GP is most likely to understand what is normal. GP's have a low false-negative rate for serious illness, or put another way they are good at finding patients who are well. Occasionally one slips through the filter, which is why GPs carry professional indemnity insurance.

The group of patients who end up being referred are thus more likely to have an illness which will benefit from specialist care than the unsorted population who consult the GP in the first place. This is crucial to the effectiveness of the referral process. The clinical methodology used by hospital consultants is primarily aimed at *detecting illness*. The sensitivity and specificity of an investigation depends on the prevalence of the disorder in the population being tested.[21] If unsorted cases are all sent off to hospital, not only would the hospitals be overwhelmed, but the false-positive rate for illness would rocket. This is no good for patients or resources.

Consider the role of the *medical test*. By convention, the range of normal for a physiological parameter is that which includes 95% of measurements in a normal population, so 5% of normal people will show abnormal on the test. The more tests are done, the more chance of one of them giving an abnormal result, so that after 20 tests a normal patient has only a one in three chance of all the results being normal'.[22]

Taking an example from malignant melanoma, one way of preventing the disease would be to remove all moles surgically, a clearly impractical suggestion. Encouraging patients to present moles they are worried about direct to dermatologists produces a very high false-positive rate: in the USA and Holland, where such open access exists, for every melanoma diagnosed there are respectively 250 and 500 benign lesions found. In Britain only 20 lesions are referred for each malignant melanoma found.[23] Experienced observers can achieve about 90% accuracy in identifying malignant melanoma,[24] but the final diagnosis can only be made by biopsy. In Britain if 10% of referred lesions are thought to be malignant, and 5% actually are, then one benign lesion is biopsied for every melanoma found. The corresponding figures for unnecessary biopsies in USA and Holland would be 24 and 49, respectively.

Exceptions

In some circumstances it is appropriate that patients refer themselves to hospital. In A&E departments *urgency* prevails. Genito-urinary medicine clinics must adopt a wider population approach than the GP list can provide for services such as *contact tracing*. The use of the emergency (999) service by the public is increasing at around 10% a year, but the proportion of these people who end up being admitted to hospital, just under half, is staying about the same.[25]

In most Western health services self-referral is the norm. In Britain the referral system was granted exemption from the Restrictive Practices Act 1976 because of its advantages to the public.[26] As the current referral system is clearly very efficient (in the sense of securing the best results from the resources available), this is deemed to take priority over the right to self-refer. However the Monopolies and Mergers Commission periodically review the situation, and so it cannot be assumed that the current arrangements for referral will exist for ever.

On the other hand patients in Britain do still self-refer to hospitals via A&E departments having previously seen their GP for the same problem.

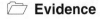 **Evidence**

> **Attending A&E for a second opinion[27]**
>
> - 20% of A&E attenders are sent by their GP
> - 10% referred themselves for a second opinion
> - The group of self-referrers had just as much chance of being admitted (28%) as other A&E attenders.

It should be remembered that the doctors in most A&E departments use consultant rather than GP methodology when deciding on an admission.

Some patients also self-refer to A&E departments with conditions which would normally be treated by GPs, but without having seen their GP first. Some will not be registered with a GP. Others will assume that a GP who has been working all day will not provide an out-of-hours service, an argument not without its sympathisers within general practice. Yet others will assume that they will get better and prompter care if they attend A&E.

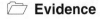 **Evidence**

> **A&E attenders with primary care problems[18,28]**
>
> A study in London found that 41% of A&E attenders had primary care problems, of whom
>
> - 10% were referred to on-call teams
> - 9% were referred to fracture clinics
>
> (Both these rates far in excess of normal GP practice)

Comparing normal A&E doctors with GPs working in the department, the A&E doctors were:

- three times more likely to refer patients to on-call teams and outpatients
- three times more likely to request radiological examination.

What are the reasons to refer?

GPs are bound by their terms and conditions of service to refer patients on to other NHS services where appropriate. The reasons for which a referral to a specialist may be appropriate are:

- Diagnosis not known
- Confirmation or exclusion of a serious diagnosis
- Necessary tests or treatment only available in hospital
- Second opinion requested by a patient
- Sharing the load of a difficult case.

🗁 Evidence

Reasons for referral[29]

According to a study from Oxford:

Diagnosis	35%
Treatment	35%
Management advice	15%
Share the load of care	10%
Patient or doctor reassurance	5%

The referral letter

This is the usual form of first contact and has potential for much more than just booking an appointment. The information included by the GP may give valuable insights into the patient, their family and social circumstances, as well as the clinical condition. Similarly the consultant's reply can be an important educational device.

📄 Guidelines

Content of a referral letter[30]

Hart and Marinker have suggested that referral letters should include:

- Clear identification of the patient
- A succinct description of the patient's personality, but avoiding caricature and character assassination
- A statement about the presenting problem
- A summary of relevant past events, including treatments tried and the patient's response
- GP's formulation of the problem
- GP's and patient's expectations of the referral
- What the patient has been told about the condition and the reason for the referral.

How good are our letters?

The content of referral letters from GPs is not as good as it might be.

 Evidence

Content of GP referral letters[31]

A study of orthopaedic referrals from Nottingham.
Items found in more than 50% of letters

- Reason for referral
- History of the problem
- The examination findings

Found in under 25% of letters

- Social history
- Family history
- Information given to the patient.

How good are the replies?

General practitioners have shown a preference for letters about their patients which are structured in so far as they contain a problem list and a list of management proposals.[32] Around 90% of letters do not meet this criterion.

The scope for education using referral letters and replies is also underused. Another study of orthopaedic referrals in Nottingham showed that items of education appeared in 3% of referral letters from GPs. Educational content was found in 26% of replies, and these replies were more likely to be written by senior registrars than by consultants or others.[33]

The referral debate

Referral to hospital is an expensive business. The wide variation in referral rate between GPs begs the question as to whether the higher referrers are wasting resources. Curiously, the corollary of this argument, whether consultants should be more efficient in their throughput of outpatients, does not seem to have had much of an airing.

A literature review in 2000 looked at 91 papers to try to identify factors that might explain the variation in GP hospital referral rates[1]

- The age, sex and social class of the patients seen by a GP explains about 25% of the referral variation observed. Other work suggests that up to a third of referral variation is explained by patient deprivation[34]
- Higher-referring GPs refer more in all clinical categories
- There is no firm association between practice size and referral rates
- If the outpatient clinic is geographically nearer there tend to be more referrals. If the waiting time for a clinic is shorter there tend to be more referrals[35]
- The personal characteristics or educational attainments of GPs do not seem to have much effect on their referral rates. The rate is not influenced by age, prescribing rate or experience in the referral specialty, except that there is some evidence that experience in a specialty actually increases the referral rate to that specialty,[36] presumably because either the GP is more aware of what benefits consultant treatment may offer, or because significant

disease is recognised at an earlier stage or because as far as that specialty is concerned the GP is still in hospital mode.

The only consistent GP factors found in surveys which differentiate between low and high referrers are:[3]

- The ability to tolerate uncertainty
- The desire not to appear foolish to consultant colleagues
- GPs who believe that serious illness occurs infrequently refer to hospital less often.[1]

It is not at all clear what the ideal referral rate is. There is a balance between conserving resources and ensuring patients get the benefit of any interventions which will help. Once a referral has been made there is a case available for examination. Patients in the group who consult their GP but who are not referred may have something to gain from specialist care, but because they are not referred there is not a case to examine. The majority of people with symptoms do not consult a doctor at all.

Are some referrals unnecessary? Most referrals have a clear medical indication, but consultants accept the vast majority of referrals as appropriate[3] either because they appreciate the problems which GP have with some patients (patients who go into a consultation with their GP expecting a specialist referral are six times more likely to be referred[37]), or because of the ability of hospital consultant clinical methods to detect pathology rather than health.

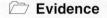 **Evidence**

Appropriateness of referrals[38]
A study of referrals to all specialties in one district health authority in the Midlands independently assessed by specialists and a GP (between whom there was broad agreement) - 13% of referrals were inappropriate - 4% of patients had been referred to the wrong specialty.

It might be that the numbers of inappropriate referrals would be higher for GPs with higher referral rates, but there is no conclusive evidence for this. There is, for instance, no evidence that cancer sufferers who present at a later stage of their disease process are more likely to have been referred by a GP with a low referral rate.[39] Practices with high referral rates also have high admission rates[1] which suggests that the hospital team in the main agree that the referrals are appropriate. The rate of referral of an individual GP is in any case difficult to define. The number of referrals is easily counted, but the denominator to the equation is more elusive

- Practice populations differ in age/sex distribution, morbidity patterns and social features
- Most GPs now work in groups, and within a group practice the patients

registered with a particular GP are often very different from the ones who are actually seen

- Doctors within a group practice may have particular skills and preferences which will attract particular types of patient. It makes more sense to look at whole practices rather than at individual doctors.

Is there scope for improvement?

The government not unreasonably finds the variation in referral rates between GPs disturbing from a financial point of view. GPs do have an interest in using resources in the most efficient way, but are also rightly concerned that a reduction in the referral rate may lead to patients not receiving services from which they might benefit.

Charges

In most health services rationing of care is achieved through charges to patients. In the NHS there are no charges, and rationing is achieved by waiting lists. Charging patients in Britain might curb referrals but there would probably have to be exemptions, just as 70% of prescriptions are dispensed to patients exempt from charges. Also, referral decisions would have to take account of the patient's ability to pay rather than concentrate exclusively on the likely benefits of referral.

Rationing

GPs might be given referral quotas. This is probably impractical because of the relatively small numbers of patients which each GP refers. A quota per specialty is even less likely to work: for some specialties a GP is likely to make a referral only once every few years. And what happens to the patients who are unfortunate enough to contract their illness at the end of the year when the quota has run out? Fixing a quota is a way of estimating what the correct referral rate is, and at present nobody has this information: it would be unjustified to fix a referral quota just on the basis of cost. However unfair the idea of a referral ration might sound, in some Primary Care Trusts individual practices are being allocated indicative referral targets, and in others practices are being urged to share their referral data with other practices.

Audits and protocols

Since the distribution of referral rates of GPs is so wide, it is impractical just to target the high referrers. The number of GPs involved in such an exercise would approximate to half of the total. In any case the effect of slightly shifting the referral habits of all GPs has a much larger total impact than picking off a few bad apples.[21]

Feedback on referrals, as long as it is ongoing,[40] would be expected to make referrals more appropriate. This can be reinforced by GPs sitting-in on outpatient clinics and by the development of referral protocols between GPs and consultants, strategies which GPs welcome.[35] A protocol might include not only the clinical situations in which a referral is appropriate, but also advice on the sort of preliminary work up which would be desirable. The National Institute for Clinical Excellence now publish and distribute regular compilations of guidance on referrals to hospital.[41] Tucked away on an inside page it says

This Guidance does not . . . override the individual responsibility of health professionals to make appropriate decisions in the circumstances of the individual patient . . .

BUT

Health professionals are expected to take it (the Guidance) into account when exercising their clinical judgement

Protocols can be a two-edged sword especially in disputes between primary and secondary care over who does what. The presence or absence of an initial work-up will affect budgeting and contracting arrangements. And who pays if an investigation, however relevant, is done more than once? What will patients and their GPs think if an agreed protocol has not been followed? Could there be medico-legal implications?

Under-referral is much harder to assess. One option is to use significant event analysis: when a problem arises with a patient, the case is subjected to analysis to find out, among other things, if a referral would have helped.

Purchaser/provider split

A central hope of fundholding was that it would make the GP/hospital interface more market orientated and hence more efficient. Fundholding made no difference to referral rates.[42] This is not surprising. Many of the initiatives taken by fundholders, in response to clear patient demand, were designed to reduce waiting times and provide satellite outpatient clinics. When patients and GPs know they are not going to be waiting a year or more for an outpatient appointment then referral becomes a useful management option. No fundholding GP wanted to be thought to be denying a patient referral in order to protect the budget.

Whether Primary Care Group/Trust commissioning will make any difference remains to be seen. Many of the initiatives being looked at to manage waiting lists have already been tried by fundholders.

Summary

- About 90% of illness presented to a doctor in the UK is dealt with in general practice
- A consultation in hospital is much more expensive than a consultation in general practice, both to the NHS and to the patient
- The present referral system in the NHS is a product of history and power-politics. However, it is incredibly efficient and the envy of the developed world
- GPs and hospital specialists solve medical problems in different ways. Subjecting an unsorted population of patients to specialist assessment would result in poorer use of resources
- Making the most of a referral requires good information exchange between GP and specialist
- Only a small part of the difference in referral rates between GPs can be accounted for by the personal characteristics of the GP

- About one in eight referrals is deemed inappropriate
- Nobody knows what the correct referral rate is
- Suggestions for altering the rate of referral all have severe limitations. The one method, fundholding, which was subjected to trial had no effect.

💬 Topics for discussion

- Patients have a right to see a hospital specialist
- A partner who refers significantly more or less than the practice average should be brought into line
- A GP should always refer to a named specialist
- Practice referral data should be shared within the PCG/T
- What are the advantages and disadvantages of auditing the practice's referral letters?
- A number of PCG/Ts are encouraging GPs to get involved in the direct booking of outpatient consultations. What might be the implications of this?

📖 References

1. O'Donnell C A. Variation in GP referral rates: what can we learn from the literature? *Fam Pract* 2000; 17: 462–71.
2. Moore A T and Roland M O. How much variation in referral rates among general practitioners is due to chance? *BMJ* 1989; 298: 500–2.
3. Metcalfe D H H. Referrals: could we do better? *Update* 1991; 42: 1093–6.
4. Hensher M and Edwards N. Hospital provision, activity, and productivity in England since the 1980s. *BMJ* 1999; 319: 911–14.
5. Anon. Record number of GP referrals. *General Practitioner* June 11 1999: 35.
6. Lydeard S. Improving outpatient visits. *The Practitioner* 1992; 236: 871–5.
7. Anon. The cost of non-attendance. *General Practitioner* November 27 1997: 4.
8. *Medeconomics* May 2001.
9. Kernick D P, Reinhold D M and Netten A. What does it cost the patient to see the doctor? *Br J Gen Pract* 2000; 50: 401–3.
10. Armstrong D and Nicoll M. Consultants' workload in outpatient clinics. *BMJ* 1995; 310: 581–2.
11. Emberton M. Outpatient follow up. *BMJ* 1995; 311: 1315–16.
12. Anon. Did not attend. *Bandolier* 1999; 6(11): 4–5.
13. Marinker M. The referral system. *J Roy Coll Gen Pract* 1988; 38: 487–491.
14. Ainsworth S. The naming of general practitioners. *General Practitioner* October 16 1998: 98.
15. Pereira Gray D. Facts and figures about general practice. Royal College of General Practitioners Members' Reference Book. London: Sabrecrown Publishing, 1991.
16. Kernick D. The Laws of Evidence-based Medicine. *Br J Gen Pract* 1999; 49: 504–5.
17. Sweeney B. The referral system. *BMJ* 1994; 309: 1180–1.
18. Dale J, Green J, Reid F et al. Primary care in the accident and emergency department: I. Prospective identification of patients. *BMJ* 1995; 311: 423–6.
19. Hannay D R. The symptom iceberg. London: Routledge and Kegan Paul, 1979.
20. Pendleton D, Schofield T, Tate P et al. The consultation. Oxford: Oxford University Press, 1984.
21. Mathers N and Hodgkin P. The Gatekeeper and the Wizard: a fairy tale. *BMJ* 1989; 298: 172–3.
22. Anon. Editor's choice: Are you normal? *BMJ* 1997; 314: 3 May.

23. MacKie R M. Clinical recognition of early invasive malignant melanoma. *BMJ* 1990; 301: 1005–6.

24. Taylor A and Gore M. Melanoma: detection and management. *Update* 1994; 48: 209–19.

25. Mann C and Guly H. Is the emergency (999) service being misused? Retrospective analysis. *BMJ* 1998; 316: 437–8.

26. Palmer K. Assessing the referral system. *The Practitioner* 1991; 235: 42–4.

27. Nguyen-Van-Tam J S and Baker D M. General practice and accident and emergency department care: does the patient know best? *BMJ* 1992; 305: 157–8.

28. Dale J, Green J, Reid F et al. Primary care in the accident and emergency department: II. Comparison of general practitioners and hospital doctors. *BMJ* 1995; 311: 427–30.

29. Coulter A, Noone A and Goldacre M. Why general practitioners refer patients to specialist outpatient clinics. *BMJ* 1989; 299: 304–8.

30. Hart J T and Marinker M. An exchange of letters. London: MSD Foundation, 1985.

31. Pringle M. Referral letters – ensuring quality. *The Practitioner*, 1991; 235: 507–10.

32. Rawal J, Barnett P and Lloyd B W. Use of structured letters to improve communication between hospital doctors and general practitioners. *BMJ* 1993; 307: 1044.

33. Jacobs L G H and Pringle M A. Referral letters and replies from orthopaedic departments: opportunities missed. *BMJ* 1990; 301: 470–3.

34. Hippisley-Cox J, Hardy C, Pringle M et al. The effect of deprivation on variations in general practitioners' referral rates: a cross sectional study of computerised data on new medical and surgical outpatient referrals in Nottinghamshire. *BMJ* 1997; 314: 1458–61.

35. McColl E, Newton J and Hutchinson A. An agenda for change in referral – consensus from general practice. *Br J Gen Pract* 1994; 44: 157–62.

36. Marinker M, Wilkins D and Metcalfe D H. Referral to hospital: can we do better? *BMJ* 1988; 297: 46–4.

37. Webb S and Lloyd M. Prescribing and referral in general practice: a study of patients' expectations and doctors' actions. *Br J Gen Pract* 1994; 44: 165–9.

38. Jenkins R M. Quality of general practitioner referrals to outpatient departments: assessment by specialists and a general practitioner. *Br J Gen Pract* 1993; 43: 111–13.

39. Hippisley-Cox J, Hardy C, Pringle M et al. Are patients who present late with cancer registered with low referring practices? *Br J Gen Pract* 1997; 47: 731–2.

40. Harris C M, Jarman B, Woodman E et al. Prescribing: a suitable case for treatment. London: RCGP, 1984.

41. National Institute for Clinical Excellence. Summary of Guidance Issued to the NHS in England and Wales. Volume 2, April 2001.

42. Illiffe S and Freudenstein U. Fundholding: from solution to problem. *BMJ* 1994; 308: 3–4.

Sleep problems

Tutorial aim	**The registrar can take a sleep history, and can manage most sleep problems within general practice.**
Learning objectives	By the end of the tutorial the registrar can:

- Discuss the relation of sleep to health
- Describe normal sleep architecture
- List the five categories causing insomnia: the *Five P's*
- Explain sleep hygiene, stimulus control and sleep restriction to a patient complaining of insomnia
- Describe the appropriate use of sedating medication
- Discuss the particular problems of sleep in the elderly
- Refer appropriately for sleep problems.

The purpose of sleep

Normal sleep is made up of two distinct components, *rapid eye movement* (REM) sleep and non-REM sleep. Non-REM sleep is further subdivided into four types

- Stage 1 is the drowsy transition from waking to sleep
- Stage 2 is the first real stage of sleep
- Stages 3 and 4 are deep sleep. Stages 3 and 4 are often called *slow wave sleep* because of the characteristic electroencephalogram pattern they produce.

Sleep architecture is the term used for the arrangement of these different types of sleep. In the normal adult sleep architecture consists of an initial period of progression through the stages of non-REM sleep, followed after about 90 minutes by the first episode of REM sleep. During REM sleep *dreams* occur. REM and non-REM sleep then alternate until waking. Episodes of REM sleep get longer, and non-REM sleep get shorter through the night: most non-REM sleep occurs in the first third of the night, and most REM sleep in the last third.[1]

- Most adults need to sleep seven or eight hours a night, but individual needs vary from four to nine hours
- Infants and children need most sleep, adults less, and there is a further decline in old age

- Growing adolescents need more sleep[2]
- There has been an 8% increase in average working hours in the last 30 years, leaving less time for sleep and recreation
- Adolescents sleep 20% less now than they did 100 years ago.[3]

In an increasingly 24-hour society, sleep is sometimes regarded as an optional extra, something to do if there is nothing better going on. Sleeping is associated with laziness: most famously, Margaret Thatcher claimed to run the country on very little sleep.

No one seems quite sure what sleep is for. It is suggested that sleep exists to comply with the theory of *conservation of energy*: wakeful activity must be balanced by a period of energy conservation while asleep, characterised by low oxygen consumption. The body's metabolic rate falls between 5 and 25% during sleep. It is also suggested that sleep has a *restorative function* for both mental and physical processes. Anabolism and catabolism are continuous processes, but when oxygen consumption is at its least, anabolism is at its peak, and there is also a surge in growth hormone release associated with non-REM sleep. Children really do grow at night. REM sleep may be more important for mental refreshment, and non-REM sleep for physical refreshment.[1]

- If sleep is either more than two hours shorter or, significantly, two hours longer than the age-adjusted norm, this is associated with an increased mortality rate in women of 68%, and in men of 29%:[3] it is as dangerous to sleep too much as too little
- Loss of sleep is associated with reduced ability to perform many tasks, particularly those which are repetitive or which require vigilance[4]
- The effects of sleep deprivation become apparent at around 18 hours, and are in many respects similar to alcohol intoxication[5]
- Sleep disruption in former shift workers can persist for 10 years after the shift work is stopped.[3]

A number of medical disorders occur more commonly during sleep or just after waking, such as coronary thrombosis, stroke, GORD, cluster headaches and sudden infant death syndrome. The peak time for all deaths is 6 am.[3] Up to 20% of all drivers have fallen asleep at the wheel, and a third of lorry accidents where the driver is killed can be attributed to fatigue.[3]

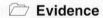 **Evidence**

Dangers of obstructive sleep apnoea[3]
 • Fallen asleep once when driving (60%) • Fall asleep once a week while driving (25%) • Increased risk of accident – between twofold and sevenfold.

The prevalence of sleep problems

Insomnia is a subjective feeling of dissatisfaction about sleep. It is important to try to pin down what a patient means when they say they are unable to sleep properly. Possibilities include

- Trouble going to sleep
- Early waking
- Broken sleep
- Duration of sleep may vary from day to day in an unpredictable way
- Fatigue in the day which is attributed to not enough sleep the night before
- Bored or unhappy with life and wish to sleep for unreasonably long periods as a means of escape from reality.

All these sleep disturbances imply different causes, and help can only be offered if the diagnosis is known.

- Around *three in ten* of all people suffer a sleep problem from time to time[6]
- When asked, about a third of people who go to see their GP, and two thirds of people who see a psychiatrist, complain that they are dissatisfied with their sleep[7]
- These figures increase with age so that over the age of 70 only half of people are happy with their sleep, a quarter have occasional problems, and a quarter are troubled often or all the time[8]
- On the other hand less than 0.5% of people with a sleeping difficulty present their problem to a GP.[3]

📁 **Evidence**

Causes of insomnia (British Sleep Society figures)[6]

Psychiatric	34%
Drugs/alcohol	16%
'Restless legs'	13%
Life circumstances	12%
Sleep apnoea	5%
Medical disorder	5%
Circadian, including shift work	5%
Perennial (childhood onset)	5%
Others	5%

Sleep is not infinitely restorative, and some people have *unrealistic expectations* of its benefits. On the other hand, there is good evidence that the correction of sleep deficiency improves daytime alertness.[8] Many human physiological variables follow a daily rhythm. *Circa* (about) and *diem* (day) are the Latin origins of the term *circadian*: these rhythms in fact run for precisely 24 hours and 11 minutes and not the variable times which were previously thought to distinguish humans from all other animals.[9]

Fatigue has a major peak about 5 am, and a lesser peak in mid afternoon. Body temperature (and oxygen consumption) is at its lowest at around 5 am, so this is when falling asleep is most likely. After this time body temperature begins to rise again whether you are asleep or not, and waking is more likely: if you go to bed late you are unlikely to stay asleep for the normal duration.

The majority, around 80%, of instances of insomnia are associated with other medical or psychiatric disorders. If sleep is to be improved, these other causes should be identified and dealt with, if possible. It may be helpful, when trying to identify the cause of a sleep problem, to recall the *Five P's*:[10]

Physical
- Cough, pain, breathlessness, tinnitus, restless legs, cramp, nocturia and paroxysmal nocturnal dyspnoea can all cause trouble getting off to sleep and/or frequent waking
- Chronic fatigue syndrome, diabetes, obstructive sleep apnoea, anaemia and hypothyroidism can cause daytime fatigue.

Physiological
- Jet lag, shift work, heavy meals or exercise before retiring, increasing age
- External noise, such as a snoring partner.

Psychological
- An acute situational crisis will commonly render sleep impossible
- Some people will worry about not being able to go to sleep, and the possible consequences of this. Such performance anxiety may escalate into a vicious circle.

Psychiatric
- Anxiety typically causes problems going to sleep. Depression usually causes early waking, but up to 20% of sufferers sleep more than normal
- Psychosis commonly affects sleep patterns
- In dementia sleep architecture can disappear altogether, giving the typical night-time wakefulness.

Pharmacological
- Non-psychotropic medications such as appetite suppressants, anti-emetics, antihistamines, corticosteroids, antihypertensives and diuretics can lead to daytime drowsiness or night-time waking
- Cimetidine, clonidine, steroids, digoxin and propranolol may cause nightmares[2]
- Low concentrations of *nicotine* are sedating, but higher levels increase arousal: smoking more than one cigarette within an hour of going to bed will cause trouble getting to sleep. The half life of nicotine is one to two hours,[11] so later wakefulness is unlikely to be due to nicotine. On average smokers sleep for 30 minutes less a night than non-smokers[11]
- *Alcohol* is a sedative, and one or two units at night will help with sleep. It is metabolised at a rate of about one unit per hour, and as levels fall to zero there may be a withdrawal effect with arousal: large amounts of alcohol can cause early waking
- *Caffeine* causes cortical arousal, and doses over 300 mg (about five cups of instant coffee) interfere with sleep. The half life is long (five hours),[11] and much longer in pregnancy,[6] so it is not just the consumption of coffee in the evening which is significant. Some people use caffeine to arouse them in the day, and alcohol to sedate them at night. Because of the different half lives, both drugs can contribute towards early waking.

Sleep hygiene
People who complain of poor sleep can often be helped by a description of the functions of sleep, and how sleep architecture develops and changes with

age. The patient's sleeping pattern may in fact be quite normal, in which case attempts to alter the pattern are unlikely to succeed.

Whether the sleep problem is due to an underlying medical condition or not, attention to what are called *sleep hygiene* measures will be of benefit.[2] The advice corresponds with the causes of insomnia given above.

📄 **Guidelines** | **Sleep hygiene[12]**

- *Exercise.* Late afternoon or early evening is best. Avoid exercise near bedtime. Fit people sleep better
- *Diet.* Snacks before bedtime should be light, and fluid intake limited. Maintain a routine
- *Caffeine.* Consumption of tea, coffee and cola should be moderated
- *Alcohol.* Regular heavy use may disrupt sleep. For sleep problems a hot milky drink is better
- *Environment.* Bed and mattress should be comfortable. Room temperature should be around 18°C (65°F). It is usually possible to adapt to noise unless it is acutely intrusive.

Psychological treatments

These can be used in conjunction with sleep hygiene measures.

- *Stimulus control* seeks to exclude the troubles of the day by making bedtime as regular and stress free as possible
- *Sleep restriction* is designed to increase the efficiency of sleep, that is to increase the proportion of the time in bed that is spent actually asleep.

The relevance of each method will depend on the patient's problems and circumstances. Problems getting to sleep are more likely to benefit from stimulus control, whereas patients who lie awake getting increasingly annoyed because they are not asleep will get more help from improving sleep efficiency. The suggested methods will take several weeks to be fully effective.

📄 **Guidelines** | **Psychological treatments for insomnia[2]**

Stimulus control

- Go to bed only when sleepy
- Use bed to sleep (no reading, eating, watching TV)
- If unable to sleep, after 10 to 20 minutes get up, leave the room, and do something else until sleepy
- Repeat above as often as necessary
- Get up at the same time each day, whatever time you went to bed
- Don't nap in the day

Sleep restriction

- Keep a sleep diary
- From the diary, estimate the average total sleep time (TST) and time in bed (TIB)

- Allow maximum TIB to be no more than average TST
- When sleep efficiency (TST/TIBx100) reaches 90% on five consecutive nights, extend TIB by 15 minutes
- Repeat above until sleep is satisfactory.

Physical tension when going to bed will result in sleeplessness. There should be a time period of at least 90 minutes before bedtime to *wind down* from the day. Some people find that controlled breathing and sequential muscle tension and relaxation are effective in reducing physical stress before retiring, techniques well established in the management of anxiety. The body is easier to relax than the mind.

📄 **Guidelines**

Reducing intrusive thoughts[2]

- Take 20 minutes each evening to reflect on the day, and consider achievements in relation to objectives. Be encouraged by achievements. Write things down
- Allocate time during the next few days to tidy up any loose ends
- Write down any other worries, decide what is the next positive step, and when this will be taken
- When in bed, refer any intrusive thoughts to the next day.

Medication

Sleeping pills have had a very bad press recently. The popularity pendulum has swung to the extent that it is assumed that all patients will be immediately addicted after one or two doses. This is not the case. The desire for more sleep is widespread. Sleep is a restoration and an escape. As such, it seems to many patients to be an obvious way out of physical, psychological and social problems.

There is no point in prescribing sleeping pills to someone whose real problem is uncontrolled pain or breathlessness, and it may prove physically dangerous to do so. On the other hand, the short-term use of sedatives can be an extremely useful way of relieving a temporary crisis, of achieving some respite until the dust has settled. As long as you keep to the restrictions given in the licences of sedatives there is unlikely to be any medical or legal problem.

At one time barbiturates seemed to be the answer, and many patients were taking them over long periods. Then the dangers of barbiturates were appreciated, and many of the same patients got moved (following considerable effort by their doctors) onto the safer benzodiazepines. Now these are no longer allowed for long-term use, and so a lot of patients have been changed onto sedating antidepressants. The problems remain; the strategies have altered.

The *benzodiazepines* are the safest available sedatives for short-term use. Half lives vary from two hours for triazolam, to 64 hours for flurazepam. Medication with a short half life is best if drowsiness the next day is to be avoided. However, a pill with a short half life may not maintain sleep throughout the night.

Temazepam has a half life of eight hours, and so is probably the most widely used sleeping tablet. It is indicated only for the short-term treatment of insomnia.[13] The covering notes in the British National Formulary suggest its use for a day or two for jet lag or shift work, and for *no more than three weeks* (preferably only one week) for insomnia associated with medical illness or emotional crisis. The point is made that tolerance can develop in as little as three to 14 days, so that the effectiveness of the medication is reduced.

Zopiclone and zolpidem have very short half lives, and do not seem (yet) to cause the dependence associated with benzodiazepines. They are much more expensive. *Chloral hydrate* is more toxic in overdose than the benzodiazepines.[2] The sedating *antihistamines* such as promethazine can be bought over the counter, but they don't work very well as sleeping pills.

Depression often causes a sleep disturbance. The typical pattern is of early waking, but in some people there is trouble getting off to sleep, and in others (especially the young) sleep is prolonged. When a sleep problem seems to have a psychological origin, it is always worthwhile enquiring after other symptoms of depression. If depression is present, then *sedating antidepressants* such as amitriptyline can be particularly useful, and all antidepressant medications should eventually help the disturbed sleep pattern. Antidepressants have not (yet) been found to have addictive potential which makes them attractive for longer-term use.

Sleep problems in the elderly

With age, normal *sleep architecture alters*. Old people need less sleep, but are more likely to complain of insomnia. One in eight of the elderly take hypnotics, the proportion being greatest for those over 70, women, and those in hospitals, nursing homes or residential institutions. The elderly are more vulnerable to the acute sedative effects of hypnotics and also to the longer-term hangover effects. An elderly person's ability to live independently may be compromised by the injudicious use of medication.

The elderly are also more likely to have *chronic pain, breathlessness,* and myriad other symptoms which may disturb sleep. They are more likely than younger people to be taking medication which interferes with normal sleep. Bereavements and depression are commoner. The risk of having a sleep-related traffic accident rises steadily from the age of 50, but interestingly there is a 'U' shaped curve so that the risk in a 90-year-old is about the same as that in a 20-year-old.[8]

Though sleep is shorter and less deep in older people so that frequent waking is common, getting off to sleep is not usually a problem. Daytime napping increases with age, and is more pronounced in men: 25% of 70-year-olds and 45% of 80-year-olds.[8] Daytime napping is probably normal, but it is also an independent predictor of death in the elderly.[14] Feelings of fatigue and tiredness in the day are often attributed to poor sleep, but are more likely to be caused by an underlying physical disorder, for example the stiffness of arthritis, the breathlessness of heart failure or COPD.

In the *elderly, there is more likely to be an underlying cause for insomnia.* The search for physical and psychological illness should be particularly careful. There may be more than one problem disrupting sleep, and treatment should be chosen which does not make things worse. The elderly are more sensitive than younger people to the adverse effects of sedatives so it is recommended to start with half the usual adult dose.

Obstructive sleep apnoea

Up to 60% of middle-aged and elderly men snore, and up to 4% of these will have obstructive sleep apnoea (OSA).[15] As the sufferer falls asleep, a loss of tone in the pharyngeal dilator muscles causes an obstruction to airflow and a choking sensation which partially rouses the sufferer.[16] This can happen up to once a minute, or 400 times through the night.[15] The sleep partner will be aware of loud snoring interspersed with episodes when breathing stops. The sufferer will experience:[15]

- Excessive sleepiness in the day
- Impaired work performance
- Morning headache
- Intellectual deterioration
- Increased risk of accidents.

Risk factors for OSA include[16]

- Male sex
- Advancing age
- Obesity
- Upper airway abnormalities
- Use of alcohol and hypnotic drugs.

If OSA is suspected, then referral to either a chest physician or an ENT surgeon is a good idea: the diagnosis is confirmed by formal sleep studies, and treatment is by the use of a continuous positive airways pressure (CPAP) machine.

Narcolepsy

Narcolepsy is a seizure disorder characterised by[16]

- Excessive daytime sleepiness (several episodes a day)
- Disturbed sleep at night
- Vivid dreams
- Sleep paralysis.

If suspected, the patient is best referred as treatment is difficult and frequently associated with troublesome side effects.

Questions to ask

- What is *meant* by 'insomnia': trouble getting to sleep, waking in the night, early waking, daytime fatigue?
- What are the *expectations* of sleep? Are they realistic?
- Has there been a *recent change* in sleep pattern?
- Is there something that is *keeping the patient awake* or waking them up (such as physical or mental symptoms, noise)?
- Is there evidence of an *undiagnosed* physical or psychological problem?
- What is the input of recreational *drugs*?

- What is the input of prescribed or over-the-counter drugs?
- What does your patient *expect* by way of treatment?

Summary

- Sleeping problems are common
- 'Not sleeping well' is an entirely subjective assessment
- Poor sleep is associated with increased morbidity and mortality
- Most people with sleeping problems do not attend their GP
- There are many possible reasons why people sleep poorly, and there is no single solution to the problem
- Sleep hygiene, stimulus control and sleep efficiency methods often work and they don't have any side effects
- Always consider depression
- A minority of patients with poor sleep have obstructive sleep apnoea, or more rarely narcolepsy
- If you want to prescribe, think first whether sleeping pills are the right approach
- If sleeping pills are the right approach, use them with confident caution.

Topics for discussion

- If you don't get enough sleep, it makes you ill
- Going without sleep is all right as long as you can catch up at weekends
- A good GP will always let his elderly patients have a few 'sleepers'
- Intelligent people need less sleep
- Should the practice run a sleep clinic? Who should staff it? What resources and training might they need? Should it be by open referral?

References

1. Shapiro C M and Flanigan M J. *ABC of Sleep Disorders* Function of sleep. *BMJ* 1993; 306: 383–5.
2. Ashton C H. Management of insomnia. *Prescribers' Journal* 1997; 37(1): 1–10.
3. Shapiro C M and Dement W C. *ABC of Sleep Disorders* Impact and Epidemiology of sleep disorders. *BMJ* 1993; 306: 1604–7.
4. Waterhouse J. *ABC of Sleep Disorders* Circadian rhythms. *BMJ* 1993; 306: 448–51.
5. Anon. Career Fous Briefing. *BMJ* Classified 21 October 2000: 3.
6. Idzikowski C. Sleep disorders. *General Practitioner* 7 October 1994: 35–41.
7. Berrios G E and Shapiro C M. *ABC of Sleep Disorders* 'I don't get enough sleep, doctor'. *BMJ* 1993; 306: 843–6.
8. Swift C G and Shapiro C M. *ABC of Sleep Disorders* Sleep and sleep problems in elderly people. *BMJ* 1993; 306: 1468–71.
9. Minerva. *BMJ* 1999; 319: 134.
10. McGhee M F. Coping with insomnia. Training, *Update* February 1998: 5–7.
11. Stradling J R. *ABC of Sleep Disorders* Recreational drugs and sleep. *BMJ* 1993; 306: 573–6.
12. Espie C A. *ABC of Sleep Disorders* Practical management of insomnia: behavioural and cognitive techniques. *BMJ* 1993; 306: 509–11.
13. British National Formulary No. 40. London: BMA/RPSGB, 2000.
14. Minerva. *BMJ* 1999; 319: 460.
15. McNicholas W. Sleep apnoea and snoring. *General Practitioner* November 6 1998: 48–9.
16. Shneerson J. Sleep disorders. *Geriatric Medicine* 1999; 29(10): 41–3.

Stroke: acute management and rehabilitation

Tutorial aims	**The registrar can appropriately assess and manage acute stroke and TIA.**
	The registrar can plan a programme of post-stroke care.
Learning objectives	By the end of the tutorial the registrar can:
	• Describe five features of acute stroke
	• Describe appropriate training for reception staff receiving a call for unconsciousness
	• Discuss the advantages and disadvantages of hospital admission
	• Describe the roles of other professionals involved in post-stroke care
	• Offer appropriate post-stroke lifestyle advice
	• Prescribe appropriate post-stroke medication
	• Help a stroke survivor and their carers to choose appropriate post-stroke follow-up.

Introduction

Stroke, or cerebrovascular accident (CVA), is defined as: 'Rapidly developing clinical signs of focal loss of cerebral function, with symptoms lasting more than 24 hours or leading to death, with no apparent cause other than that of vascular origin'.[1]

A transient ischaemic attack (TIA) is defined as: 'An acute loss of focal cerebral function with symptoms lasting less than 24 hours with no apparent cause other than that of vascular origin'.[2]

Each year in the United Kingdom there are:[3]

• 110 000 first strokes
• 30 000 recurrent strokes
• 10 000 strokes occurring in patients under 55
• 60 000 deaths from stroke[4] (representing 12% of all deaths and making stroke the third commonest cause of death[5])

Stroke is more likely to occur in patients who have had a previous episode: after a CVA the risk of *recurrence* in the first year is 13%, and in subsequent years 5%.[5] The overall incidence of stroke is 2 per 1000 per year. Putting this into primary care terms, an *average GP* will have four new strokes a year to deal with, as well as 12 to 15 patients who have survived a stroke.[5]

- Over the past 20 years there has been a *reduction in mortality* from stroke of between 2% and 7% each year.[5] The beginning of this reduction predates the widespread interest in treating hypertension
- Twenty four per cent of the *severely disabled* in a community are stroke victims[6]
- Stroke care consumes around 5% of all NHS *resources*,[1] about £2.3 billion a year[7]
- In addition, 25 000 people a year suffer a *TIA*.[8]

What to do when called to a possible stroke

It is important to *attend promptly*. The onset of a stroke usually causes great distress because the symptoms are often severe and dramatic and come on quickly. Stroke is commoner in the hours just after waking,[9] so the call often comes before or during the morning surgery.

The suddenness of onset implies a vascular cause for the symptoms, and a diagnosis of stroke is even more likely if there are known risk factors. Ninety per cent of strokes affect the cerebral hemispheres, and of these 75% occur in the territory of the internal carotid artery and 15% in the vertebrobasilar artery territory (in the other 10% the picture is not clear).[2]

Carotid territory stroke typically causes:

- Hemiparesis and facial paresis
- Monocular visual loss
- Dysarthria
- Dysphasia (dysphasia of language if the dominant hemisphere is involved, or visuo-spacial dysphasia if the non-dominant hemisphere is involved)
- Conjugate gaze to the side of the lesion
- Homonymous hemianopia.

Vertebrobasilar stroke may cause much less obvious bilateral symptoms:

- Bilateral blindness
- Homonymous hemianopia
- Diplopia and nystagmus
- Problems with gait and stance
- Vertigo
- Hemi- or bilateral motor paresis
- Hemi- or bilateral sensory loss
- Dysarthria.

Stroke is by a long way the commonest reason for the sudden onset of a neurological deficit in an elderly person, but other possibilities should also be borne in mind.

📄 Guidelines

Differential diagnosis of stroke[4]

- Decompensation of previous stroke
- Cerebral neoplasm (progressive symptoms)
- Subdural haematoma: after head injury
- Epileptic seizure
- Brain trauma
- Migraine
- Multiple sclerosis
- Cerebral abscess.

Clinical examination

The clinical examination should be to confirm the diagnosis of stroke and to exclude alternatives.

- *Neurology* Consciousness level will give an indication of the severity of the stroke, and so the likelihood of recovery. Other objective localising signs (such as hemiparesis) will help to confirm the diagnosis
- *Blood pressure* More than half of stroke victims have hypertension.[10] Stroke causes BP to rise acutely and then fall again over several days. Any decision to lower blood pressure should be delayed for at least 10 days after the stroke[11]
- *Heart rate and rhythm* About one in twelve stroke sufferers have atrial fibrillation[10]
- *Heart sounds* The presence of a valvular lesion may suggest that anticoagulation or surgery might be considered
- *Peripheral pulses* Nearly a quarter of stroke victims have peripheral vascular disease. Of particular interest is the presence of a carotid bruit which suggests (but does not confirm) significant stenosis. If stenosis of more than 70% is present, then carotid endarterectomy reduces the risk of further stroke by 75% over three years.[12]

Admission to hospital

The National Service Framework (NSF) for Older People identifies stroke as its fifth standard for care. It recommends that people with suspected stroke should usually be admitted urgently to hospital.[3] Given the weight of evidence in support of this recommendation it is difficult to think of situations in which urgent hospital admission would not be desirable. However, if symptoms are very mild and there is patient objection, or if symptoms are so severe that death is imminent, then there is probably an argument against admission. Currently about 80% of stroke victims get admitted to hospital,[13] but this varies in different parts of the country so that in some areas around half of cases are kept at home. Stroke patients account for 12% of general medical and 25% of geriatric bed-days.[14]

- *Specialised stroke care* improves the short- and long-term outlook for sufferers.[15] Community rehabilitation is better than no care or day hospital.[16] Specialised inpatient care from a dedicated *multidisciplinary team* is better than non-specialist care at reducing disability and shortening hospital stay, but even so 60% of stroke victims are either dead or dependent one year after their stroke.[15] By 2004 all stroke victims are to have access to a specialised stroke unit.[3]

- Four fifths of strokes are caused by ischaemia. Treatments for ischaemic stroke are not a good idea in haemorrhagic stroke, and presently the best way of distinguishing the two is by *brain imaging* which has to be done within 14 days of the vascular event.[1] CT scanners are found in hospitals. The short- and long-term prognosis is worse after haemorrhagic stroke.[4] The NSF has supported the recommendation of the Royal College of Physicians guidelines on stroke care[17] that all patients with stroke should have a brain scan within 48 hours.[3]
- Ischaemic stroke causes the death of neurones, but not straight away. The few hours after onset are the most important. In the US routine use of thrombolysis is recommended within three hours of stroke,[15] and where the US leads we will surely follow. The future may bring neuroprotective medication. In Britain the place of such treatments is not established. However, it remains true that the maintenance of oxygenation and blood chemistry will *promote neurone survival*: medical stabilisation is urgent, and most readily achieved in hospital.[17]
- The psychological effects of a stroke on the victim and their carers are commonly very severe. Many patients and families find a hospital admission of *psychological benefit* over and above any improvement in morbidity or function.[18] It acknowledges the severity of the event, and removes the need of the carers to decide whether or not they can cope.

Patients who have suffered a TIA should be referred urgently to a rapid response neurovascular clinic.[3] By definition the symptoms of a TIA can go on for up to 24 hours, but it is recommended that hospital admission is needed if:[4]

- Symptoms have persisted for more than an hour
- There is a second TIA within a week
- A TIA occurs in a patient who is already receiving anticoagulants.

After a stroke

Answering patient questions

The outlook after a stroke is not very good. Patients and their carers are entitled to accurate information, however distressing this may be. Creating unrealistic expectations causes more problems in the long run.

Death

- The patient suffering a stroke will have a 30% chance of dying within the first month after it.[3] Of these deaths, half will be due to the acute effects of the stroke and half due to complications, for example pneumonia[1]
- Ten years later a stroke victim has only a one in two chance of still being alive. Fifteen per cent will suffer a subsequent fatal stroke, but 40% will die of a myocardial infarction.[19] Stroke is only one manifestation of vascular disease.

Disability

- Eighty per cent of surviving stroke victims live in the community, but 25% are entirely dependent on a carer, and a further 30% need help with daily living tasks. Hence less than half of stroke victims end up being fully independent[20]
- After six months, 50–80% of patients will be able to walk independently but only 22% can walk at their previous speed[21]
- Around 25% of stroke sufferers become depressed.[22] This is about twice the level of the normal elderly population (at 15%), and is about the same as for other elderly people with a chronic debilitating illness. The site and extent of the cerebral damage does not correlate well with the chance of depression.

Recurrence

- After a stroke, the victim has a 13% chance of recurrence in the first year, and 5% per year thereafter.[5]

Secondary prevention

Following a stroke the risk of death is raised. If a stroke has occurred it means that there exists significant vascular pathology. The risk of subsequent death through a heart attack is greater than that of death from a further stroke. Risk factors should be attended to where appropriate. Patients with the greatest risk levels have the most to gain from preventive measures.

Hypertension should be brought under control gradually. After a stroke, there is a linear relationship between the risk of a further stroke and both diastolic and systolic blood pressures: each 5 mmHg lower diastolic pressure is associated with a 34% decreased risk, and each 10 mmHg lower systolic pressure with a 28% decrease.[23] This is the same order of benefit as is seen in lowering blood pressure in the primary prevention of stroke; but since people who have already had a stroke are at much greater risk of having another, the benefit per stroke patient of lower blood pressure is much greater. The target pressure for secondary prevention of stroke should be less than 130/80 in diabetics and less than 140/85 in non-diabetics.[24]

Elderly patients are at greater stroke risk, and so potentially have more to gain from treatment. Treating hypertension in the very old has yet to demonstrate benefit conclusively, but there is clear advantage to be gained up to age 80.[25]

Smoking should be counselled against, and offers made to help smokers to stop.

A *low fat diet* is reasonable advice, though the protective value of cholesterol-lowering drugs is unsure.[1]

Aspirin. Following a stroke, the risk of future vascular events can be reduced by about a quarter by treatment with aspirin. The non-fatal myocardial infarction and stroke rate is reduced by a third, and the rate of vascular death is reduced by one sixth.[26] The benefit is only seen in patients who have had an ischaemic stroke: following haemorrhagic stroke, aspirin should not be used. An initial dose of 300 mg followed by daily doses of 75 mg is advised.[24] Benefit has been demonstrated from continuing aspirin treatment for up to two years. It is probable that the benefit is continuous, and so the indefinite use of aspirin is recommended.[26] *Clopidogrel* is an alternative, albeit an expensive one, in patients unable to take aspirin.

Modified-release *dipyridamole* 200 mg bd is as effective as aspirin in secondary prevention, and has an additive effect with aspirin.[24]

Anticoagulation with warfarin keeping the international normalised ratio (INR) between two and three is recommended after a stroke in patients with atrial fibrillation.[24]

Tertiary prevention

The stroke patient who is admitted to hospital will usually be discharged after an average of two to three weeks, during which time there will have been an intensive rehabilitative effort. It is important that discharge be *properly planned* so that community support structures can be set up. Close liaison between hospital and primary care in all disciplines is vital. The NSF recommends that stroke victims and their carers should have access to a *stroke care coordinator* after discharge.[3]

It is suggested that recovery from a stroke goes through four stages[27]

- Crisis
- Treatment
- Realisation
- Adjustment.

Hospitals tend to concentrate on the first two of these. This can lead patients and carers to the belief that this is the only form of treatment available. Despondency results when it is evident that a degree of disability will persist.

Intrinsic Recovery, the return of neurological function, occurs over the first three months only. *Functional recovery*, the ability to do things, occurs by a combination of intrinsic recovery and adaption. The full process may take up to 12 months, with 5–10% of the improvement happening in the later six months. Further improvement after 12 months is very unlikely.[21]

There is a need for realistic information and explanation so that other ways of minimising disability can be looked for at an early stage. The NSF recommends that a stroke victim who still has *significant disability at six months* should be offered a *further assessment* and further targeted rehabilitation.[3]

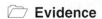 **Evidence**

Awareness of prognosis after stroke[20]
In a study from general practice, 65% of spouses were still expecting the full recovery of the patient 16 months after the stroke.

Stroke rehabilitation: the GP's role

Access to services

An early assessment should be made, and community services mobilised if this has not already been done. Secondary preventive strategies initiated in hospital should be reinforced. The GP also has a *gatekeeper role* to provide the patient with access to other services.

📂 **Evidence**

Access to stroke services[13]
A study reported in 1993 that at three months after discharge • One third of stroke victims had still not seen their GP • 27% had had no inpatient physiotherapy • 67% had had no out-patient physiotherapy.

Information

Informed and realistic information and advice are needed by the patient and their carers. This can be supplemented by the excellent literature available from the Stroke Association (previously part of the Heart Chest and Stroke Association).

> The Stroke Association
> Stroke House,
> Whitecross Street
> London EC1Y 8JJ
> Tel: 020 7490 2686

A discussion of prognosis is appropriate. Advice on resumption of normal activities can be useful, especially with relation to *sexual activity*: only a third of patients return to their previous levels of sexual activity after a stroke.[21] Advice on eating, smoking and alcohol may be needed.

Driving is not advised for a month after a stroke.[28] The vehicle licensing authority (DVLA) will need to be informed if a stroke has occurred. If the victim is left with epilepsy, substantial motor or visual loss or significant sensory inattention, driving should not be resumed. If there is *doubt about driving ability* the DVLA can arrange an independent medical examination and a formal driving test. Modifications to the car may be made.

Symptom control

Depression is very common among stroke victims. It should be specifically looked for as it will respond to antidepressants in standard doses. Bear in mind that the average stroke victim will be elderly and the stroke indicates that there is *significant vascular pathology*: if urinary retention or cardiac arrhythmia is likely, then the newer antidepressants with fewer side effects can be useful. It is usually wise to begin with a small dose with a view to later increase.

Depression should be distinguished from *emotionalism* which also frequently accompanies a stroke. The patient may become weepy and distressed for no obvious reason, to their embarrassment and the distress of their carers. Emotionalism may show some response to antidepressants.[22] In general, emotionalism is best seen as a type of illness behaviour, and care must be taken by carers and professionals that the behaviour is not inadvertently reinforced.

Pain, in particular shoulder pain, may be present. Spastic muscles are prone to spasm. Muscle and even bone injuries may occur. Pressure areas need regular review. Pain may respond to simple analgesia such as paracetamol 1000 mg six hourly, or to ibuprofen 400 mg eight hourly if there is an inflammatory element to the pain and there are no contraindications.

In addition, stroke sufferers may get *central post-stroke pain* (CPSP or thalamic syndrome). This affects between 2 and 6% of victims and is commoner in younger patients. The onset of symptoms is commonly delayed for several weeks or months after the stroke. An area of burning pain is felt, often associated with autonomic instability and *allodynia* (the feeling of pain following non-painful stimuli). There is invariably an area of sensory loss to pinprick which extends beyond the bounds of the pain.[29]

The pain of CPSP does not result from the stimulation of pain fibres, it is a result of damage to the cerebrum. Because of this, standard analgesics, however powerful, often do not work. Nortriptyline and amitriptyline in standard antidepressant doses will help, but they do not have a licence for use in pain relief. Clinical response takes four to six weeks.

Information on *insomnia* and *incontinence* may not be volunteered unless enquired after. *Leg swelling* and *contractures* in the affected limbs will be visible on clinical examination. *Pressure sores* and *fractures* are commoner in the stroke victim. *Falls* are more common after a stroke. The maintenance of balance requires the adequate function of the balance-maintaining senses (proprioception, sight, vestibular function); the ability to correct minor degrees of imbalance so that a stumble does not become a fall; and the ability centrally to integrate the balance information. The brain deficit following a stroke may impair central integration and reduce the patient's ability to correct a stumble.[30] In addition, because of the age of the average stroke victim, they will probably already have some impairment of the other balance systems.

Psychological support

Problems of psychological adaption will be present to a greater or lesser extent in all stroke survivors. Communication difficulty with speech or language, receptive or expressive, will benefit from the involvement of a speech therapist. Impaired mobility may benefit from aids and adaptions and modified transport. The occupational therapist is an invaluable resource. Dependency and boredom are almost universal among stroke victims. Very few patients readily adapt their hobbies to their disabilities and will tend to dwell on what they cannot do rather than on what they can do.

Dealing with Crises

The two major crisis points are at the time of the stroke, and on discharge from hospital. The withdrawal of active therapy may give a sense of rejection.

If the carer becomes ill or dies, or there is an additional health problem such as a fracture, then the whole care plan has to be rethought.

Supporting the Carers

Most of the care of stroke victims in the community is done by informal carers. The majority of these are spouses, and so usually elderly themselves. Next in order of frequency are daughters and daughters-in-law.

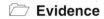 **Evidence**

> **Health of stroke carers[20]**
>
> - 14% of carers will have given up work to look after the stroke victim
> - 12% of stroke carers are depressed, and this figure is 40% in the case of spouses. The patient's wife is more likely to be depressed than the patient.

Financial advice is often needed. Some benefits are particularly relevant to the stroke victim, such as the *Attendance Allowance* and, for those under age 65, the Disability Living Allowance. Further advice can be obtained via advice centres or social workers.

Respite admissions and day care can give the carer a well-earned rest. The Stroke Association, other voluntary bodies and many hospital stroke units provide *stroke clubs* for the support of patient and carer, but these facilities are often not known about.

Transient ischaemic attack (TIA)

A TIA is the same as a stroke in all respects of definition, except that the symptoms resolve completely within 24 hours. *Amaurosis fugax* is a transient monocular visual loss lasting under 24 hours (and usually a couple of minutes only). This and TIA are due to small emboli which in 75% of cases arise from the internal carotid artery.[2]

There are 25 000 TIAs a year in the UK, an incidence of one per 1000 or two per average GP list. Having a TIA increases the risk of a subsequent stroke in the next year thirteenfold,[8] and 15% of strokes are preceded by a TIA.[2]

The diagnosis of TIA may be difficult as there are many other reasons why patients have dizzy spells. In one series only a third of patients referred to a clinic with a diagnosis of TIA had been correctly diagnosed.[2]

The risk factors for TIA are the same as those for stroke. When a TIA is diagnosed or suspected then an early cardiovascular and cerebrovascular assessment is needed. Aspirin 75 mg a day can be started unless there are contraindications.

Summary

- Stroke is a leading cause of death and disability in the United Kingdom, even though its prevalence is falling
- Nearly all stroke victims benefit from inpatient assessment and rehabilitation
- After a stroke the patient will get better for about a year, and there will be little improvement thereafter

- After a stroke a patient is more likely to die of a heart attack than from another stroke
- A stroke has psychological as well as physical consequences
- Stroke carers often make themselves ill through their duties
- Most stroke victims and their families are financially disadvantaged.

✎ Topics for discussion

- A patient suffering a stroke should ring an ambulance without contacting their GP at all
- The treatment of raised blood pressure in patients over age 80 is likely to be of benefit
- Patients discharged from hospital after a stroke should routinely be visited by their GP
- What are the advantages and disadvantages of giving warfarin to more patients?

📖 References

1. Sandercock P A and Lindley R I. Management of acute stroke. *Prescribers' Journal* 1993; 33: 196–205.
2. Naylor A R and Bell P R F. Management of mild symptomatic CVD. *Update* 1993; 47: 670–5.
3. National Service Framework for Older People. London: DoH, 2001.
4. Bath P M W and Lees K R. *ABC of arterial and venous disease.* Acute stroke. *BMJ* 2000; 320: 920–3.
5. Dennis M and Warlow C. Strategy for stroke. *BMJ* 1991; 303: 636–8.
6. Greveson G and James O. Improving long-term outcome after stroke – the views of carers. *Health Trends* 1991; 23: 161–2.
7. Fowler G. Stroke: The general practice perspective. *Geriatric Medicine* 1999; 29(12): 30–1.
8. Naylor A R. Carotid endarterectomy for the prevention of ischaemic stroke. London: The Stroke Association, 1993.
9. Wroe S J, Sandercock P, Bamford J et al. Diurnal variation in incidence of stroke: Oxfordshire community stroke project. *BMJ* 1992; 302: 155–7.
10. Forbes C D. Secondary prevention of stroke and TIA. *Targeted Therapeutic News* No. 45, July 1999.
11. O'Connell J E and Gray C S. Treating hypertension after stroke. *BMJ* 1994; 308: 1523–4.
12. Brown M M and Humphrey P R D on behalf of Association of British Neurologists. Carotid endarterectomy: recommendations for management of transient ischaemic attack and ischaemic stroke. *BMJ* 1992; 305: 1071–4.
13. Crowe S. Stroke prevention: More than just monitoring BP. *Monitor Weekly* 1993; 6(22): 41–2.
14. Young J. Is stroke better managed in the community?: Community care allows patients to reach their full potential. *BMJ* 1994; 309: 1156–7.
15. Management soon after a stroke. *Drug and Therapeutics Bulletin* 1998; 36(7): 51–4.
16. Young J B and Forster A. The Bradford community stroke trial: results at six months. *BMJ* 1992; 304: 1085–9.
17. Wade D and the Intercollegiate Working Party for Stroke. London: Royal College of Physicians, 1999.
18. Pound P, Bury M, Gompertz P et al. Stroke patients' views on their admission to hospital. *BMJ* 1995; 311: 18–22.

19. Marshall J. Why patients at risk of stroke should take aspirin. *Monitor Weekly* 1994; 7(13): 43–4.
20. Cassidy T P and Gray C S. Stroke and the carer. *Br J Gen Pract*, 1991; 41: 267–8.
21. Hewer R L. Stroke-induced disability. *Update* 1994; 48: 375–85.
22. House A. Depression after stroke. *BMJ* 1987; 294: 76–8.
23. Rodgers A, MacMahon S, Gamble G et al. Blood pressure and risk of stroke in patients with cerebrovascular disease. *BMJ* 1996; 313: 147.
24. Lees K R, Bath P M W and Naylor A R. *ABC of arterial and venous disease.* Secondary prevention of transient ischaemic attack and stroke. *BMJ* 2000; 320: 991–4.
25. Ramsay L E, Williams B, Johnston G D et al. British Hypertension Society guidelines for hypertension management 1999: summary. *BMJ* 1999; 319: 630–5.
26. Underwood M J and More R S. The aspirin papers. *BMJ* 1994; 308: 71–2.
27. Forster A and Young J. Stroke rehabilitation: can we do better? *BMJ* 1992; 305: 1446–7.
28. Driving after a stroke or TIA. London: The Stroke Association, 1994.
29. Bowsher D. Central post-stroke pain and its treatment. London: The Stroke Association, 1994.
30. Overstall P W. Falls after strokes. *BMJ* 1995; 311: 74–5.

Terminal care at home

Tutorial aim	**The registrar can manage a terminally ill patient in the community.**
Learning objectives	By the end of the tutorial, the registrar can:

- List all the stages of a loss reaction
- Describe five considerations when delivering bad news
- List three ways of improving team communication, where the team includes carers
- Help a terminally ill patient and their carers to contribute to a programme of palliative care
- Describe the analgesic ladder
- Discuss social and personal attitudes towards death
- Maintain appropriate confidentiality.

Statistics

Around 23% of people in the United Kingdom die at home and 71% in institutions: 54% in hospital, 13% in nursing or residential homes and 4% in hospices. At the beginning of the century the vast majority of deaths occurred at home.[1] Because people are living longer, more people die when they are elderly. Twenty five per cent of people live alone,[1] and this group are mainly elderly. Lack of family support is an important reason why people do not die at home.

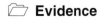 **Evidence**

Preferred place of death[2]

Of people who are expecting to die

- About half would rather die at home
- A quarter would rather die in hospital
- A quarter would rather die in a hospice.

If home circumstances had allowed, two thirds of the sample would have expressed a preference to die at home.

In 1993 the Institute of Actuaries estimated that the *cost of caring* for the elderly and disabled was £40 billion (£52.6 billion at 2000 prices) a year, and set to rise to between £60 billion and £100 billion a year by 2033. Three quarters of the cost is borne by lay carers and a quarter by the state.[3]

A third of cancer patients receive care from just one relative, while a further half are cared for by two or three relatives, typically a spouse and an adult child.[4] As the average age of death gets later, so the age of carers goes up: over 50% of carers are above retirement age.[5]

📁 **Evidence**

Where is terminal care conducted?

In their final year of life[1]

- 75% of people spend under three months in hospital,
- 54% spend under a month in hospital
- 16% spend no time in hospital at all

On average, 47 weeks of the last year of life are spent at home.[6]

Even for those who die away from home, much of the terminal care still falls onto community resources. The primary healthcare team deal with 90% of palliative care needs.[7]

A GP with an average list size will have about five patients each year who die at home. In addition there will be at any one time around two patients who are terminally ill and at home.[6]

Malignant disease accounts for only 3.5% of primary care cases,[6] but the workload generated by each case tends to be high. Death can be predicted with some confidence months or occasionally years after diagnosis. Death from non-malignant disease is less predictable, and occurs on average between one and nine days after diagnosis.[8]

The psychology of the terminally ill

When a terminal diagnosis is made, there will be a sense of loss: loss of health, loss of faculty and loss of a future. The stages of the grief reaction are the same as for a bereavement.

- Numbness
- Pining
- Disorganisation and despair
- Reorganisation.

Nine tenths of cancer sufferers *want to be told their diagnosis*, exact details of their illness and what treatment options are available.[9] Four fifths want as much information as possible, and a fifth are dissatisfied at the amount of information they receive.[10] Patients must have access to sufficient information to be able to make informed choices about their care and their future. In addition, sharing information about an illness, even if the prognosis is poor, may give the patient more hope for the future.[11]

The pining stage of grief is commonly associated with powerful outbursts of anger and distress. Such emotions are inevitable and a normal part of the grief process. Suppression of emotion hinders the grieving process, but the patient's distress may make bystanders wonder if confirming the terminal diagnosis was indeed the best strategy.

Depression is also a normal part of a grief reaction. In addition, the terminally ill will usually be disabled, and sometimes in pain: it is not surprising that around 50% show evidence of depression.[6]

The final phase, reorganisation, can take several months, and may not be completed before death.

The psychology of the carers

The lay carers of the terminally ill at home are *almost always close family members*. The making of the terminal diagnosis will also have an impact on them. Not only will they have to contend with their own grief, they also face the physical and psychological demands of the dying person.

Many carers will try to put on a brave face. This is partly a form of denial, but is rationalised as an act of kindness, a way of relieving the patient's emotional burden. Many carers sustain their brave face with remarkable tenacity, but later are faced with the double burden of their delayed grief and the emotional and physical exhaustion consequent on their caring duties. *Terminal care is care of the carers as much as care of the patient.*

Conspiracy of Silence

Carers are generally less willing than doctors to be open about a fatal diagnosis and to discuss death.[8] Carers may affect jollity and false optimism. The patient usually reacts by thinking that the carers are unable to face up to the imminent death and so they also try to make believe that they are not expecting to die. At the time when family relations need to be at their closest, things are clouded by lies and deceptions. Encouraging the open discussion of feelings and fears is an important aim for the GP.

Sometimes family members will insist that the terminal diagnosis is not disclosed to the patient. They may feel unable to cope with the force of the emotions such a disclosure will inevitably provoke. They may feel that the patient will give up and hasten their death. They may feel that they are in some way offering protection from upset. These fears are not borne out by the available evidence. It is commonly family members who are less involved in caring who will forbid disclosure, whereas those more closely involved are able to see how much strain is caused by restricting communication.

🗎 Guidelines

Withholding a terminal diagnosis

The doctor's role is very clear: while respecting that the family know the patient best, it is ethically wrong to tell lies. Confronted with a direct question from a patient about their condition, a doctor is obliged to offer a truthful answer.

Carers gain most satisfaction from their duties when they are *involved* explicitly and continuously.[12] Doctors are not very good at predicting when death will occur, tending to overestimate prognosis:[13] unrealistic estimates of how long their work may go on can be received with mixed emotions by carers.

The psychology of the professionals

Coping with terminal illness creates emotional problems for the professionals involved, as well as for the patient and their family. The professionals may not have worked through their own feelings about death, and may have unresolved grief of their own. They too are affected by the general social taboos which surround death.

In addition the professionals bear a burden because of the responsibilities of their role.

- In general, people enter the caring professions because they want to help. Delivering bad news and upsetting people does not come easily
- The emphasis in medical training is on curing. A terminal diagnosis is a failure, a sign of professional inadequacy
- Coping with the emotional demands of the dying requires high quality communication skills, skills which medical schools have only recently begun to teach. There may be a fear of being blamed, of not knowing the answers or of saying and doing something which will make things worse.

However, medical and nursing specialists in palliative care tend to have lower rates of anxiety and depression than their colleagues, possibly because of the professional satisfaction which terminal care can bring.[4] Training clearly has a protective effect.

Inverse confidentiality

Once a fatal diagnosis has been made, professionals tend to go into terminal mode. The emphasis changes to palliation and there is less concern about drug dependency etc. Any patient not already aware that they are dying will almost certainly realise that a change in tactics has occurred. The GP may end up giving more information to the carers than to the patient, a sort of inverse confidentiality where the patient actually knows less about their condition than does their family. This cannot be condoned, but is perhaps understandable. Many professionals have difficulty in discussing such sensitive issues with terminally ill patients. In addition the GP will quite rightly appreciate the important role which lay carers play, and this in itself requires that the carers are given full and accurate information.

The team

If terminal care at home is to be successful, *the patient's family must be welcomed as members of the primary healthcare team*. Carers have their own needs: half will be suffering from anxiety and over a third will be depressed, even though half find their caring duties rewarding and only 10% find them a burden.[4] They will have valuable insights into the patient's condition and state of mind, insights likely to be more accurate than those of the attending nurses and doctors. They bear the brunt of the caring duties and should be accorded the same professional respect as other team members.

- Lay carers are not given the support they should expect from the professional carers
- A known carer who attends the surgery should not be kept waiting around for longer than is necessary

- Special provision should be in place to respond to carers' enquiries, e.g. telephone access to the responsible doctor: good teamwork thrives on good communications
- Each terminal care contact should include consideration of the welfare of the carers.

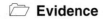 **Evidence**

> **Support for carers[14]**
>
> - 70% of carers spend seven or more hours a day in their caring duties
> - 90% have not been given advice about lifting and handling techniques
> - only 14% report that their GP had visited to see how they were managing.

Two thirds of cancer patients receive visits from the district nursing team.[4] District nurses provide the most regular contact with the patient and their family, and can usually be regarded as team leaders in the terminal care situation. The *Macmillan service*[15] is funded by the National Society for Cancer Relief. Macmillan nurses all have district nurse or health visitor training, and then additional specialist training. They are involved with about 40% of cancer patients[4] and their contribution to the physical and psychological needs of the dying patient and their family can be considerable. It is not uncommon for terminally ill patients to be reluctant to bother the GP with their symptoms. Macmillan nurses encourage open discussion of death and dying, and their realistic approach to the benefits of palliative care creates a more relaxed and honest therapeutic environment. However, care must be taken to make sure that the existing doctor/district nurse team is not disrupted by the new expert.

Breaking bad news

There is a long tradition of doctors telling lies to their patients. In 1672 the French physician Samuel de Sorbiere considered the idea of telling patients the truth, but concluded that it could seriously jeopardise medical practice and so would not catch on. In 1961, a survey of American surgeons found that 90% would not routinely discuss a diagnosis of cancer with their patients.[16]

The evidence that patients want, benefit from and are entitled to more information about their medical condition, even if the prognosis is poor, is now unassailable. This has caused a sea change in the attitudes of doctors: by 1979, 90% of American physicians would routinely discuss a diagnosis of cancer, but this change was driven by the patients' right to truth enshrined in American law rather than because doctors decided it was medically desirable. British doctors have lagged behind: in 1985 between half and three quarters of British GPs and consultants would not routinely disclose a diagnosis of cancer.[16]

Even so, doctors do not like giving their patients bad news. They too may fear the patient's immediate reaction, and share a sense of professional failure that the disease is incurable. In addition, the doctor may not be quite sure what bad news is. Bad news is: '*The discovery that reality is going to fall short of expectations*'.[9] What those expectations are can only be known by the patient. The meaning of a loss can only be understood by the person who is undergoing it.

When a fatal diagnosis is suspected, confirmation by a specialist will usually be arranged. A *second opinion* should be encouraged for those patients who wish it.[9] This may lead to confusion over who is responsible for telling the patient the bad news. It is vital that there is early feedback after a specialist consultation including details of what the patient and their family have been told. Consultants may have their own hang-ups about breaking bad news, but the disclosure of a fatal diagnosis is clearly the responsibility of the first doctor to confirm that diagnosis. Failure to discuss a terminal diagnosis may strain future relations between the GP and consultant.

Breaking or sharing bad news is an *ongoing process*. The patient and their family can take in only a limited amount of information on one occasion There may be denial so that the facts have to be gone over again. The questions to which the patient wants answers may only emerge over time. Part of palliative care is the regular review and clarification of the medical facts, and the creation of regular opportunities to discuss the implications of the terminal disease process.

What to say

The majority (up to 80%) of cancer sufferers want to be actively involved in decisions about their treatment. However only 10% of patients wish to take the major role,[9] presumably so that they are protected from the responsibility for a bad decision. In general patients who are younger, better educated and female are more likely to want to be involved. The desire to participate in management decisions is associated with greater optimism about outcome.[9]

In order to make informed decisions, the information necessary includes

- The nature of any treatment proposed, including the frequency and reversibility of any adverse effects and the expected benefits
- The duration of treatment and time in hospital
- Any non-physical effects (e.g. depression, loss of libido, family effects).

Involving patients actively in decisions about their treatment means that their wishes are complied with as far as possible. This may have the result that the patient opts for no treatment. Later in the course of a terminal illness the occasional patient will, though rational, refuse treatment or indeed food and drink because they have decided that they have had enough.[8] Euthanasia and suicide are still illegal in Britain, but on these occasions the line separating what is and is not ethical is indeed blurred.

How to say it

The communication of the fatal diagnosis has to be done carefully. The illness and any medication being taken may cause confusion.

'*We are brought up not to lie, especially in professional life – but equally we know that how we handle the telling of truth is crucial*'.[17]

Information has to be specific and concrete. The words used should be understandable. When breaking bad news, the following may help:[18,19]

- *Set the scene*. Make sure all the medical details are at hand. Who does the patient want present? Is there enough space, enough chairs? Make sure there is enough time: it will always take longer than the doctor thinks/ hopes. For the GP a home visit will usually offer greater flexibility.

- *Check the background.* How much do the patient and family already know? This can be done by asking them to tell you what has been happening
- *Check what is wanted.* In a minority of cases the patient may not want to know any more, but this should be distinguished from the patient who is afraid to ask for more information
- *Start gently.* Preface the discussion by saying that the news is not very good
- *Go slowly.* Don't try to deliver the information too quickly. Pause between pieces of information. Does the patient want you to go on?
- *Expect the worst.* Some patients will respond with denial, others with anger and others with acute distress. All these are normal, but hard work to handle
- *What are the worries?* Try to find out what the patient's immediate concerns are. These may be predictable, such as fear of dying or pain. Others are less predictable, and can only be found out by asking
- *Encourage the ventilation of feelings.* This is probably the part which the patient will *value most* later
- *Summarise.* Reviewing what has been said makes sure you and the patient are on the same wavelength. Make suggestions about an initial management plan, and make sure the patient agrees
- *Be accessible.* As well as planned review, it is important that the patient and their family know how to get hold of you in case of problems.

Written material or a tape recording of the consultation can be taken away for further reference.

Palliative care

Palliative care is defined by the World Health Organisation (WHO) as: *'The active total care of patients whose disease is not responsive to curative treatment'.*[20] This emphasises the active component of the care. Curative treatments need not be suddenly switched to palliative ones: the process is better seen as a gradual shift in emphasis from one to the other.

- In 90% of cases where palliative care is needed, the primary diagnosis is of cancer[20]
- Around half of GPs feel that they could benefit from further training in palliative care[21]
- Most terminally ill patients have several symptoms: the average is seven[22]
- Doctors *tend to underestimate* the quality of their patients' lives, and also underestimate the severity of their symptoms[23]
- In addition, doctors have *different priorities*: doctors have more regard to physical function and less regard to social function and pain than do their patients
- The concordance between carers and patients is better than between patients and doctors in estimating the quality of life and the severity of symptoms.[24]

Generally, patients with advanced cancer are *more likely than their doctors expect*, and more likely than healthy people, to opt for major but possibly curative procedures even though there is a risk of severe toxicity and the possible benefits are small. In choosing treatment options patients are much influenced by what they believe their doctor wants them to do. When explaining options it is important for doctors not to let their own feelings influence the way in which information is presented.

📂 **Evidence**

How good is terminal care?[25]

Care rated 'good' or 'excellent'	89% of patients, 91% of carers
GP and district nurse care rated 'good'	71% of patients and family
Hospital services: 'good'	less than 50%
'poor'	23%

The standards of care provided by acute wards in hospitals give rise to particular concern. In an observational survey in Scotland, there was a tendency for nurses and doctors to spend less and less time caring for terminally ill patients as death became more imminent. In some cases patients were ignored on ward rounds, and basic nursing needs were neglected.[26] When specific problems are looked at, the areas still causing concern to terminal patients and their families are:[5]

- Communication, especially at diagnosis
- Coordination of services
- Attitude of doctors
- Delay in making the diagnosis
- Problems getting doctors to do home visits
- Lack of financial advice.

It will be noticed that symptom control does not appear on this list. In a 1992 MORI poll of terminally ill cancer sufferers, only 3% felt that they needed more prompt surgical care but 24% felt in need of more counselling.[27] It is a priority for the GP to ensure that the patient and their carers receive the necessary psychological support.

Respite care

Respite care for the terminally ill can be provided by hospitals or a hospice (if available). The well-timed use of a respite admission may make all the difference between the carers' ability to cope or not.

Hospitals may only accept respite patients reluctantly. Such an attitude is inappropriate and short sighted. A brief admission and a treatment sort out, with attention to nutrition, fluid balance and skin care will often reduce the subsequent need for acute care when either the patient's state or the exhaustion of the carers provokes an emergency admission.

Hospices are charitable organisations, and so according to current regulation at least half of their running costs have to be provided by charitable donations. They will accept patients on an inpatient or a day-patient basis, as well as providing terminal care advice (often through Macmillan nurses). The emphasis is on the active dimension of palliative care. More patients would wish to spend their terminal illness in a hospice rather than in hospital.

Benefits

Lack of advice about possible financial support is a common worry among the dying and their carers.

1. The *Attendance Allowance* is the benefit most often relevant to the terminal care situation. Eligible persons must be dependent on others for their bodily functions either by day, or by day and night. There is no means test. In order to qualify, the disability has to have been present for six months. This is clearly inappropriate in a terminal care situation and can be waived by use of the *Special Rules* provision, where the GP fills in form *DS 1500* attesting to the terminal nature of the illness. The attendance allowance is not meant to be a payment to the carers for their work. It is designed so that care can be bought in to help out and give the other carers a rest. The *Disability Living Allowance* is the same as the attendance allowance in most important respects, but applies to patients under 65.
2. The *Invalid Care Allowance* may be applied for if a carer under pension age has had to give up paid employment to fulfil caring duties. In addition there are a number of national and local charities which may help with voluntary or paid carers, or the provision of information and equipment. The district nursing team will usually have a good idea of what is locally available.

Euthanasia

The word *euthanasia* means a 'good death'. The law is quite clear: killing people is illegal and attracts punishment. The situation where death occurs as a side effect of treating a disease or symptom is far less clear. Treatments primarily designed to combat serious symptoms, e.g. opiates, are widely used in terminal care, and the correct dose is that which controls the symptom. If this is a fatal dose, it is still unlikely to interest the police. To be legal the intention has to be symptom control, rather than to cause death.

The British Medical Association report on euthanasia[28] concluded that it wished euthanasia to remain illegal. However the withholding of treatment from a terminally ill patient (for instance antibiotics for a terminal chest infection) was regarded as acceptable. In practice a patient who is about to die is unlikely to respond to antibiotics anyway.

In Holland, a mechanism has been in place for some years to allow the termination of life by doctors when there is no chance of recovery, where symptoms are uncontrollable and where the patient asks for it. It is estimated that 2% of the deaths occurring in general practice are assisted in this way.[29] The law in some parts of America now allows for physician-assisted suicide in some circumstances.[30] In Britain up to 90% of people would support euthanasia in the most desperate cases.[31]

The *Advance Directive* or *Living Will* is a mechanism by which people may express their feelings about life-salvaging treatments should they become terminally ill and mentally incompetent. There has been no change in UK law to accommodate the advance directive.[32] However legal opinion and case law is accumulating which supports the view that an advance directive, if it exists and is known about, is binding. A further discussion of the advance directive can be found in the notes on dementia.

Symptom control

Control of pain

- Eighty per cent of cancer sufferers experience pain.[33] Studies done in the 1960s indicated that the pain of terminal illness was not well controlled by GPs. Later work suggests that the situation is much improved with 96% of patients having their pain controlled.[5] Even so only 12% of cancer sufferers die with no pain at all.[7]
- There may be more than one type of pain, needing more than one type of analgesic. About 50% of patients will be experiencing three or more different types of pain.[6]

Pain is often constant and serves no useful purpose. Analgesic regimens should seek to be continuously effective.

The analgesic ladder
This is the approach recommended by the WHO. Control is achieved by choosing treatment from one of three groups of drugs, according to the severity of the pain. It is no good switching to different preparations in the same group if pain is not controlled; a drug from a stronger group is needed.

- *Step 1*: Mild pain can be relieved by aspirin 600 mg four hourly, or paracetamol 1 g every four to six hours. These agents may also be added to other regimens as needed
- *Step 2:* Moderate pain needs weak opioid preparations such as codeine 30–60 mg four hourly (maximum 240 mg in 24 hours), or dihydrocodeine 30 mg four hourly. Larger doses confer little extra analgesia, but increase side effects. Laxatives should be routinely prescribed
- *Step 3:* Severe pain needs narcotic analgesia of the strong opiate class. The correct dose is that which works – there is no maximum.

Morphine is the oral preparation of choice at step 3. In liquid form it is easily ingested and dosage can be titrated accurately. If taste is a problem, Oramorph (Boehringer Ingelheim) has the morphine taste masked.

🗎 Guidelines

Oral opiate use in terminal care

- At first use morphine every four hours
- Increase the dose by 50% each time until pain control achieved

- When the pain is controlled the total daily morphine dose can be given in two modified release doses, with additional morphine as needed (example: 20 mg morphine every four hours is equivalent to 60 mg modified release morphine twice a day).

Diamorphine is much more soluble and so is more suitable if *injected opiate* is needed: 1 g of diamorphine can be dissolved in 1.6 ml of water whereas 1 g of morphine requires 20 ml.[34] By dose diamorphine is between three and four times more powerful than morphine.[35]

Daytime drowsiness, dizziness and mental clouding are common at the start of treatment but *usually resolve* in a few days. Once the dose is stable, effects on cognitive and psychomotor functioning are minimal. Up to two thirds of patients when started on morphine get nausea and vomiting, but this too usually resolves. It may be appropriate to coprescribe anti-emetic agents when morphine treatment is initiated.[34]

When used appropriately to treat the pain of terminal illness the weight of evidence suggests that morphine does not cause addiction, excessive sedation or respiratory depression.[34]

Many patients will be aware that opiates such as morphine are only used in terminal care situations. This may lead to reluctance to accept the treatment, as if starting morphine hastens death. The acceptance of the terminal diagnosis may be incomplete and need further discussion.

Difficult pain

Used optimally, morphine will achieve control of pain in 80% of cancer sufferers.[34] The remainder will need other interventions. Pain arising from tissue damage is transmitted through nerve pain fibres and is termed *nociceptive pain*. It responds very well to opiates. Other types of pain may, however, be present with or sometimes without nociceptive pain. Bone pain and neurological pain do not respond well to ordinary analgesics of whatever potency.

- *Bone pain* will often respond to local irradiation or non-steroidal anti-inflammatory preparations
- *Neurological pain* will benefit from tricyclics or anti-epileptics
- *Visceral pain* responds poorly to morphine, and indeed may be made worse.[35] Laxatives will ease pain from constipation. In addition antispasmodics such as hyoscine may well help
- *Sympathetic pain* is a dull or burning sensation which is hard to localise. The painful area also shows signs of sympathetic overactivity such as erythema and sweating. Anti-epileptic drugs can be useful.

It is possible to augment the effect of analgesics with *tricyclic antidepressants* in doses up to and including those needed for depression. The pain-relieving properties of tricyclics are independent of the antidepressant properties, and may become apparent within two or three days.[6] A significant number of the terminally ill are depressed anyway, and this symptom may also be helped. Antidepressants and anti-epileptics are not licensed for use in pain control.

Route of administration

Medication should be given *orally where possible*. When this is not possible because of nausea or intestinal obstruction, then other routes have to be found. Injections are painful, particularly in the emaciated patient. Lack of muscle bulk and circulatory failure may make absorption unreliable. Many analgesics are available in the form of *suppositories*, and this is a very efficient route of delivery. Examples include morphine and diclofenac. However suppositories can be difficult to self-administer and can be ineffective if they induce reflex defaecation. Unlike in some countries, the rectal route has never been usual or popular in British medical practice. A patch delivering strong analgesic (fentanyl) transdermally became available in 1995.

Syringe driver. This is an electrical or sometimes clockwork device which slowly delivers a dose of medication over a period of time. A syringe driver cannot be prescribed, but many practices have their own as it is a popular piece of equipment for communities to donate to their local primary care services. Otherwise they can sometimes be borrowed from hospitals or hospices, or bought by the practice. A syringe driver is simply a different means of delivering medication, and has no magical properties. A subcutaneous needle is used, preferably a butterfly needle. The needle can be left in until there is evidence of blockage or inflammation at the site (up to two weeks), whereupon the infusion should be resited.

- The most suitable drug to use is diamorphine
- The 24-hour dose can be worked out by taking the amount of morphine taken by mouth and dividing it by three to get the equivalent dose of diamorphine
- The nauseating effects of diamorphine can be reduced by adding haloperidol or cyclizine to the infusion
- The normal principle of using different sites for different drugs does not apply when using a syringe driver in terminal care[36]
- Drugs which can be mixed with diamorphine include cyclizine, haloperidol, hyoscine and metoclopramide: the British National Formulary (BNF) gives details on the practical issues of mixing drugs.[36] The product liability implications of mixing drugs in this way can be defended by reference to the BNF section on terminal care.

Control of other symptoms

Nausea

Over 40% of terminally ill patients suffer nausea.[6] This may be due to the disease process or the treatment. Haloperidol is probably the medication of choice,[33] in a dose of up to 10 mg over 24 hours. Alternatives are metoclopramide, cyclizine and the phenothiazines. Causes of nausea such as *constipation, hypercalcaemia, raised intracranial pressure and intestinal obstruction* may be helped by symptomatic medication, but attention to the underlying cause is also needed.

Constipation

All terminally ill people are liable to constipation because of immobility and because constipation is a side effect of all the stronger analgesic preparations. Over 35% of terminally ill patients suffer constipation.[6] Even patients not eating need to void the cells sloughed off the bowel mucosa. Laxatives should be started as soon as strong opioids are prescribed. Stimulant laxatives or stimulant plus softener are best. Senna and bisacodyl are good stimulants. Lactulose and ispaghula husk are good softeners. Docusate has both actions. Constipation is a particularly trying symptom for the terminally ill. If no other way can be found, it is justified to use regular enemas to prevent constipation.

Diarrhoea

Faecal impaction is the commonest cause of diarrhoea in the terminally ill. Having excluded this, loperamide is probably the medication of choice.

Cough

Respiratory infections will cause cough and these may be treated with standard antibiotics. Even if the infection is secondary to bronchial obstruction by the neoplasm, treatment is the same. Cough due to wheeze may benefit from bronchodilators and steroids, but care must be taken not to provoke dyspepsia. For cough without remediable cause, steam inhalers or nebulised saline or lignocaine can help loosen tacky secretions and provide relief. Simple linctus or codeine or pholcodeine linctuses are also worth a try.

Mouth problems

Eighty per cent of patients with terminal cancer have xerostoma (dry mouth), and in 75% of cases candida is present.[37] Ice or pineapple chunks are helpful. Antifungal treatment with nystatin or amphotericin can be considered. Patients who have a dry mouth as a result of radiotherapy or sicca syndrome can have artificial saliva products prescribed under Advisory Committee on Borderline Substances (ACBS) regulations. Suitable products are Glandosane (Fresenius) and Salivix pastilles (Thames).

Depression

It is not unusual for terminally ill patients to become depressed, and this tendency is greater if other symptoms are not controlled. Around half of terminally ill patients are depressed.[6] A process of psychological support needs to be started as soon as the fatal diagnosis is made.

- It is inappropriate to be optimistic about the long-term outcome in the terminally ill
- Taking time to provide explanations about what is happening can demystify the illness and make it easier to come to terms with
- It is important to find out specifically if the patient has fears about dying. There is some evidence that death itself is quite without physical or emotional pain.[38] Patients can also be assured that every effort will be made to keep the terminal illness as free of symptoms as possible

- Specific enquiries about symptoms may reveal problems which the patient did not want to trouble you with. Good symptom control is important for psychological well-being.

If a major depression has occurred, then there is often a good response to standard antidepressant medication. Lesser degrees of depression respond less well to treatment. The fact that the patient has good reason to be depressed does not matter: if the symptoms of depression are severe then there should be a good response to antidepressant medication.

People involved in long-term informal *caring* duties have poorer health than average. Depression may well feature in their reaction to the imminent death, and should be actively looked for. The support of the caring team is an important function for the GP, and applies to lay carers as well as to the professionals.

Confusion

Around 30% of the terminally ill suffer confusion.[6] The cause of the confusion may be the illness or the treatment. Haloperidol, diazepam, chlorpromazine and chlormethiazole may be considered in the disturbed or toxic.

Anorexia

Anorexia occurs in nearly 60% of the terminally ill.[6] Dietary advice may be needed. An appetiser, traditionally sherry, may be helpful. Small portions should be offered and the patient should be tempted to eat rather than bullied.

Liquid foods will be easier to take. If food is to be liquidised, it should be shown to the patient before it is processed so that some sense can be made of the uniformly brown pulp which the patient eventually gets to eat. Proprietary brands of liquid food are also available and these can be useful. A number of them can be prescribed under ACBS regulations for the malnutrition associated with chronic disease.

Sometimes steroids help to promote the appetite in a nonspecific way. They do not, however, cause weight gain other than by fluid retention.[39]

Fungating tumours

The smell of a fungating tumour is a constant reminder of the inevitable. A course of metronidazole can be very useful to help the smell. Charcoal dressings or local radiotherapy to reduce tumour bulk are worth considering.

Immobility

Stiff joints and weak muscles are inevitable consequences of immobility. Exercises and passive movement may be suggested by the physiotherapy team. Changing the position of the patient, either actively or passively, will reduce the burden on the skin and avoid pressure sores.

Summary

- Two thirds of people want to die at home, but under a quarter manage to do so

- Most of the care of the dying at home is provided by informal carers, usually family members
- Presented with a terminal diagnosis, a patient will undergo a grief reaction much like that seen with bereavement. There may not be time before death to complete the process
- Anger and depression may be alarming to bystanders, but are a normal part of a grief process
- Carers use up their time and often their health on their duties. They should be accorded appropriate respect as key members of the primary care team
- Care of the terminally ill is frequently professionally rewarding. Professional carers will often have to come to terms with their own feelings through the work
- Carers often end up knowing more about the illness than does the patient: inverse confidentiality
- Bad news should be broken slowly and carefully. Encouraging a patient to be emotionally explicit is probably the most important component
- The pain of terminal care is managed much better than it used to be. A syringe driver is only another delivery system, and is no more effective than what the doctor prescribes to put in it.

✎ Topics for discussion

- Euthanasia will eventually be legal in Britain
- All patients should die at home if possible
- Death is not a nice subject for conversation
- Terminal care should be left to trained specialist teams
- What happened the last time you had to break bad news to a patient?

📖 References

1. Thorpe G. Enabling more dying people to remain at home. *BMJ* 1993; 307: 915–8.
2. Townsend J, Frank A O, Fermont D et al. Terminal cancer care and patients' preferences for place of death. *BMJ* 1990; 301: 415–7.
3. Tonks A. Community care fails the frail and elderly. *BMJ* 1993; 307: 1163.
4. Ramirez A, Addington-Hall J and Richards M. *ABC of palliative care*. The carers. *BMJ* 1998; 316: 208–11.
5. Jones R V H, Hansford J and Fiske J. Death from cancer at home: the carers perspective. *BMJ* 1993; 306: 249–51.
6. Sandars J. Palliative care: a GP's perspective. *Update* 1994; 48: 345–51.
7. Cox I G. Palliative care *Update* 2000; 60: 396–403.
8. Blackburn A M. The elderly dying patient. *Update* 1995; 50: 434–42.
9. Patient choice in managing cancer. Drug and Therapeutics Bulletin 1993; 31: 77–9.
10. Jones R, Pearson J, McGregor S et al. Cross sectional survey of patients' satisfaction with information about cancer. *BMJ* 1999; 319: 1247–8.
11. Eastaugh A N. Breaking bad news. *Update* 1996; 53: 8–16.
12. Minerva. *BMJ* 1999; 319: 794.
13. Christakis N A and Lamont E B. Extent and determinants of error in doctors' prognoses in terminally ill patients: prospective cohort study. *BMJ* 2000; 320: 469–73.
14. Wise J. Carers are ignored by the NHS. *BMJ* 1998; 316: 1765.

15. Brown A. The Macmillan service. *Medical Dialogue* 1985 No. 70.
16. Buckman R. Talking to patients about cancer. *BMJ* 1996; 313: 699–700.
17. Higgs R. When it's time to stop. *Update* 1998; 56: 656–8.
18. McLauchlan C A J. Handling distressed relatives and breaking bad news. *BMJ* 1990; 301: 1145–9.
19. Bodner A. Palliative care. *Update* 1996; 53: 18–23.
20. Finlay I and Forbes K. Symptom control in palliative care. *Update* 1994; 48: 180–8.
21. Haines A and Booroff A. Terminal care at home: perspectives in general practice. *BMJ* 1996; 292: 1051–3.
22. Sandars J. Palliative care: action plan. *Update* 1994; 48: 355–6.
23. Rothwell P M, McDowell Z, Wong C K et al. Doctors and patients don't agree: cross sectional study of patients' and doctors' perceptions and assessments of disability in multiple sclerosis. *BMJ* 1997; 314: 1580–3.
24. Gregor A and Cull A. Radiotherapy for malignant glioma. *BMJ* 1996; 313: 1500–1.
25. Higginson I, Wade A and McCarthy M. Palliative care: views of patients and their families. *BMJ* 1990; 301: 277–81.
26. Mills M, Davies H T O and Macrae W A. Care of dying patients in hospital. *BMJ* 1994; 309: 583–6.
27. The social impact of care in Great Britain. MORI Health Research, 1992.
28. British Medical Association. The Euthanasia Report. London: BMA, 1988.
29. Sheldon T. Euthanasia law does not end debate in the Netherlands. *BMJ* 1993; 307: 1511–2.
30. Churchill L R and King N M P. Physician assisted suicide, euthanasia, or withdrawal of treatment. *BMJ* 1997; 315: 137–8.
31. Wise J. Public supports euthanasia for most desperate cases. *BMJ* 1996; 313: 1423.
32. Davies J and Beresford D. The Advance Directive. Medical Defence Union Journal 1991; 4: 92–3.
33. Mersey Regional Drug Information Service and the Department of Pharmacology, University of Liverpool. Care of the dying. Drug information letter. MeReC, 1991.
34. Expert Working Group of the European Association for Palliative Care. Morphine in cancer pain: modes of administration. *BMJ* 1996; 312: 823–6.
35. O'Neill W M. Pain in malignant disease. *Prescribers' Journal* 1993; 33: 250–8.
36. British National Formulary No 41 (March 2001). London: BMA/RPS, 2001.
37. Jobins J, Bagg J, Finlay I G et al. Oral and dental disease in terminally ill patients. *BMJ* 1992; 304: 1612.
38. Waine C. Terminal Care. Royal College of General Practitioners' Members' Reference Book. London: Sabrecrown, 1988: 176–80.
39. Davis C L and Hardy J R. Palliative care. *BMJ* 1994; 308: 1359–62.

Urinary tract infection (UTI) in adults

Tutorial aims	**The registrar can distinguish uncomplicated from complicated urinary tract infection in adults. The registrar can manage uncomplicated urinary tract infection in the community.**
Learning objectives	By the end of the tutorial the registrar can: • List three clinical features of upper UTI • List three clinical features of lower UTI • Recall a differential diagnosis for dysuria and frequency • List criteria for *complicated* UTI • Choose appropriate further investigations • Choose an appropriate prescription • Choose with the patient an appropriate strategy for recurrent UTI.

Introduction

- One in five women will have an episode of dysuria and frequency in a given year,[1] and half at some time in their life[2]
- Episodes are commoner in the sexually active aged 20 to 50, in the pregnant, the elderly and diabetics[2]
- Only half of episodes are presented to a doctor,[3] but even so dysuria and frequency account for up to 3% of all GP consultations,[2] and 6% of consultations with women aged 15 to 44.[3]

Dysuria and frequency are much less common in men, with an incidence only a fifth of that found in women.[4] It is extremely rare in younger men but becomes commoner in the sixth decade and beyond, this increase with age being attributable to bladder outflow obstruction consequent on prostatic enlargement.[5]

Asymptomatic bacteriuria can be found 2% of women aged 20 to 50, in 10% of women aged 65 to 70,[6] or up to 50% of those who live in an institution.[5] It appears to cause no harm.[6] Up to 20% of institutionalised elderly men are also affected.[5]

Making the diagnosis

📄 **Guidelines**   **Symptoms of urinary tract infection[2]**

Lower UTI:	Dysuria
	Urinary frequency
	Urgency
	Nocturia
Upper UTI:	Fever
	Malaise
	Nausea
	Loin pain

Most women who present to their GP with symptoms of lower UTI will be issued a prescription without further ado, and will get better. Everyone is happy. However some will not get better, especially those in whom the diagnosis of UTI is incorrect.

- Only half of women presenting with dysuria and frequency have a demonstrable UTI[2]
- Half of non-pregnant women with proven bacteriuria will be better inside three days without drug treatment.[2]

📄 **Guidelines**   **Differential diagnosis of dysuria and frequency**

Women:	Lower urinary tract infection
	Urethral syndrome
	Atrophic vaginitis
	Vaginal infection, including *Chlamydia*
	Bladder stone
	Trauma – honeymoon cystitis
	Pelvic inflammatory disease
Men:	Lower urinary tract infection
	Urethritis – sexually transmitted disease
	Bladder stone
	Prostatitis

A *clinical examination* in women is unlikely to be fruitful. Loin pain may suggest an upper UTI, and abdominal palpation can be helpful. Some specialists suggest a routine vaginal examination,[7] but this view is not supported by others[2] unless vaginal pathology is suspected from the history.

In *men*, UTI is rarer and more likely to be the result of renal tract abnormality. Examination of the abdomen (for loin pain and palpable bladder), testes, epididymis and prostate may be appropriate.[4]

The use and abuse of the MSSU

A midstream sample of urine (MSSU) is one collected after the first 10 ml or so of urine have been discarded. A lower urinary tract infection exists when bacteria are actively multiplying in the bladder.[8] *Significant bacteriuria* is said to be present when 10^5 or more bacteria can be seen per ml in an MSSU.[5] This threshold, the *Kass criterion*, was first suggested in 1956 and has not changed since.

📁 **Evidence**

Sensitivity of MSSU[9]

Probability that bacteria are replicating in the bladder

One positive MSSU	80%
Two positive MSSUs	95%

- The risk of contamination of an MSSU (as suggested by the presence on culture of multiple types of bacteria) is minimised when the woman holds the labia apart before collecting the specimen.[9] Cleaning the perineum is unnecessary[10]
- In men with clinically normal genitals, no preparation is needed before voiding[4]
- The specimen should be cultured within two hours, or 24 hours if stored at 4°C. The addition of 1.8% boric acid to the MSSU stops organisms multiplying and white cells lysing, so that the specimen stays useable for several days at room temperature[9]
- The use of a dip-slide means that culture is started straight away, but makes it impossible to do any cell counts.

The result of an MSSU culture takes a minimum of two working days to acquire. Though in widespread use, the *Kass criterion is not beyond criticism*.

- The Kass criterion was developed using women who did not have cystitis[6]
- Urinary frequency lowers bacterial counts by dilution, rather as Kass predicted
- In men contamination of an MSSU is less likely so that lower bacterial counts may well be significant, i.e. 10^3 bacteria per ml[4]
- Unusual organisms, or fastidious ones that are difficult to culture, may be a significant finding at levels below 10^5 per ml.[5]

If an MSSU has been done and given a result confirming the presence of a UTI, then a repeat should be done after treatment to confirm cure.

📄 **Guidelines**

Reasons to send an MSSU

- Diagnosis not sure
- Recurrent or persisting symptoms
- Pregnancy
- Known or suspected renal tract abnormality
- Diabetes

- Significant haematuria
- Loin pain and/or systemic disturbance
- Male patient.

In suspected UTI a quicker result can be obtained by dipstick testing.

📁 **Evidence**

> ### Correlation of dipstick urine tests and MSSU[10]
>
> - The presence of urinary nitrites on dipstick testing has a positive predictive value of 89% that an MSSU will be positive, and a negative predictive value of 79%
> - The presence of urinary leukocytes on dipstick testing has a positive predictive value of 66% that an MSSU will be positive, and a negative predictive value of 90%.

Managing dysuria/ frequency

The dangers of the inappropriate use of antibiotics are well documented. In half of women who present with dysuria/frequency it is not possible to find a UTI. This may result from the deficiencies of dipstick and MSSU testing, or may be because no infection is present. Where dysuria and frequency exist but neither a UTI nor any other cause for the symptoms can be found, the woman is said to have *urethral syndrome*.[10]

The cause of urethral syndrome is not known, but there are a number of theories. It is suggested that the presence of lactobacilli in the vagina can cause dysuria and frequency.[11] Lactobacilli are hard to culture and may not appear on an MSSU. Crucially, the presence of lactobacilli is more likely when the normal vaginal flora have been suppressed by, for instance, treatment with antibiotics: the use of antibiotics for dysuria/frequency may accordingly make symptoms worse. The only thing wrong with the lactobacilli hypothesis is that they are no less likely to be present in women who have urethral syndrome than they are in women who do not, and their eradication with suitable treatment does not seem to resolve the symptoms.[12] The jury is still out.

Guidelines[2] suggest the separation of UTI into *simple* and *complicated*.

📄 **Guidelines**   **Simple *and* complicated UTI[2]**

Simple UTI is dysuria/frequency in:

- Women aged 20 to 50
- Lower UTI symptoms only
- Not pregnant
- Not diabetic
- Symptoms not recurrent (not four or more episodes a year)
- No known renal tract abnormality

Complicated UTI is everything else.

Symptomatic measures may help in all cases of UTI. Pain and fever can be helped by *analgesics* such as paracetamol 1 g qds. Some will find a *hot water bottle* useful. *Altering the acidity* of the urine with bicarbonate of soda added to drinks may relieve symptoms.[2] Drinking lots of fluid is normally recommended, but the value of this is disputed.[2]

Managing simple UTI

- If the dipstick urine test is positive, three days of *trimethoprim* 200 mg bd
- Most infections respond clinically
- Longer courses are no more effective
- Single doses work, but the rate of recurrence is increased[10]
- Trimethoprim does not affect the combined *oral contraceptive pill*[13]
- *Cephalosporins* have a similar range of activity, but are more expensive and more likely to disrupt gut flora
- *Nitrofurantoin* is also effective and does not disrupt gut flora: it may cause nausea.

An MSSU need only be taken if symptoms do not resolve after three days. If the dipstick urine test is negative, look for alternative reasons for the symptoms.

Managing complicated UTI

An *MSSU* should be taken, and a *seven-day* course of antibiotic treatment begun while waiting for the result[2]. In *men*, the responsible organisms are usually the same as for women, as is the choice of suitable antibiotics.[2] If symptoms are due to prostatitis, then antibiotics for 30 days are needed.[4]

📄 Guidelines

Referral of men with proven UTI[4]

Urology referral is required in all men with proven UTI as 70% of these will have a renal tract abnormality,[7] most commonly bladder outflow obstruction in the elderly group.

In *elderly women*, the typical symptoms of UTI may be absent, or only elicited by specific questioning. Organisms may be unusual, and so treatment is best informed by an MSSU.

Patients with symptoms of *upper UTI* (pyelonephritis) can be treated with a quinolone or co-amoxiclav for at least seven days.[2]

In *pregnant women* the prevalence of asymptomatic bacteriuria is as high as 7%:[6] nearly a third of these progress to pyelonephritis, and there is an increased risk of midtrimester abortion, premature labour and intrauterine growth retardation.[2] In pregnancy cephalosporins and nitrofurantoin appear to be safe, but trimethoprim is not. Follow-up with repeated MSSUs is needed for the rest of the pregnancy.

Guidelines

Case finding UTI in pregnancy[2]

- All pregnant women should routinely have their urine cultured at their first antenatal appointment
- Bacteriuria should be treated even in the absence of symptoms
- Follow-up is by repeated cultures throughout the pregnancy.

Patients with an *indwelling urinary catheter* will, if tested, usually have bacteriuria. Treatment is not necessary unless there is systemic disturbance or an MSSU grows *Proteus*.[14]

A patient who is severely unwell because of a UTI requires admission to hospital.

Managing recurrent UTI

- Four or more episodes of dysuria/frequency in a year, at least one of which has produced a positive MSSU, defines recurrent UTI[10]
- Patients with recurrent simple UTI should be referred to hospital to have their renal tract radiologically investigated[10]
- If the renal tract is normal, recurrence may be due to *sexual activity*. Gel can be used if lubrication is a problem. Emptying the bladder and a perineal wash down (front to back) after sex may help. A single dose of trimethoprim 200 mg after coitus can prevent an attack of UTI
- Atrophic vaginitis can cause dysuria, and also predisposes to UTI. Topical oestrogen cream may help.

In the absence of any of the above, and after confirmation that the renal tract is normal, prophylaxis against UTI may be secured by daily use of a small dose of antibiotic (e.g. trimethoprim 100 mg at night), and by the use of self-help measures.

Guidelines

Self-help in recurrent UTI[15]

- Wear cotton underwear
- Wipe front-to-back after micturition/defaecation
- Drink plenty, but limit caffeine and alcohol
- Void regularly, and ensure the bladder is empty: 'double micturition'.

Summary

- The use of dipstick tests for nitrite and/or leukocytes makes the rational use of antibiotics in UTI more likely
- The use of the MSSU has limitations
- All pregnant women should have an MSSU done at first antenatal attendance. If bacteria are found they should be treated even in the absence of symptoms
- Simple UTI needs only three days of antibiotic. Complicated UTI needs at least seven days of antibiotic
- There are many other causes for dysuria and frequency as well as UTI

- Urethral syndrome should only be diagnosed when all other possibilities have been excluded
- All patients with complicated UTI need further investigation.

✿ Topics for discussion

- Urinary tract infection is caused by a lack of hygiene
- Urinary tract infection should be regarded as a sexually transmitted disease, and treated accordingly
- It is inappropriate to expect a patient to pay £1 a tablet for trimethoprim
- Simple UTI is best managed by the practice nurse
- Dysuria/frequency is never a medical emergency.

📖 References

1. Waters W E. Prevalence of symptoms of urinary tract infection in women. *Br J Prev Soc Med* 1969; 23: 263–6.
2. Urinary tract infection. MeReC Bulletin 1995; 6: 29–32.
3. Thomas M, Kyi M and Moorhead J. Cystitis and pyelitis: urinary tract infections in women. *Maternal and Child Heath* 1990; 15: 340–4.
4. Dhillon G. Urinary infections in men. *Update* 1998; 56: 871–4.
5. Wilkie M E, Almond M K and Marsh F P. Diagnosis and management of urinary tract infection in adults. *BMJ* 1992; 305: 1137–41.
6. Brooks D. Management of cystitis. *Update* 2000; 60: 492–5.
7. Shah J. Cystitis: treat quickly, and suggest hygiene precautions. *The Practitioner* 1998; 242: 698–702.
8. Brooks D. Acute dysuria and frequency in women. Update 1995; 51: 269–74.
9. Mead M, Prentice M B and Nicholson K G. Midstream urinary investigation. *Update* 1994; 48: 155–8.
10. Managing urinary tract infections in women. *Drug and Therapeutics Bulletin* 1998; 36(4): 30–2.
11. Maskell R. Antibacterial agents and urinary tract infection: a paradox. *Br J Gen Pract* April 1992; 42: 138–9.
12. Brumfitt W, Hamilton-Miller J M T and Gillespie W A. The mysterious "urethral syndrome". *BMJ* 1991; 303: 1–2.
13. Miller D M, Helms S E and Brodell R T. A practical approach to antibiotic treatment in women taking oral contraceptives. *J Am Acad Dermatol* 1994; 30: 1008–11.
14. Khot A and Polmear A. Practical General Practice, 3rd edn. Oxford: Butterworth Heinemann, 1999.
15. Van Shaik S and Cranston D. Urinary tract infections in adults. *Update* 1996; 53: 412–16.

Useful Websites

Tutorial 1
Alcohol problems   www.alcoholconcern.org.uk
                          www.downyourdrink.org

Tutorial 2
Anxiety   anxiety.mentalhelp.net
Stress   www.healthnet.org.uk/news/stress/index.htm

Tutorial 3
Childhood abdominal pain gut1.peds.uiowa.edu/educate.htm
Attention deficit disorder www.simsue.force9.co.uk
Autism   www.oneworld.org/autism_uk
Bullying   www.successunlimited.co.uk/stress/trauma.htm

Tutorial 4
Benign prostatic
  hypertrophy   www.bui.ac.uk/noflashindex.htm
Prostate cancer   bjach.polk.amedd.army.mil/7/cancer2.htm

Tutorial 5
Breast cancer   www.cancerbacup.org.uk

Tutorial 6
Child abuse   www.yesican.org
                          www.geocities.com/Heartland/meadows/9312/
                             info.htm
                          www.nspcc.org.uk

Tutorial 7
Accident prevention   www.babyworld.co.uk/information/baby/safety/
                             garden.htm

Tutorial 8
Chronic fatigue syndrome www.smd.kcl.ac.uk/cfs
ME   www@afme.org.uk

Tutorial 9
Atheroma   www.hgcardio.com/periph.htm

Tutorial 10
Dementia   dementia.ion.ucl.ac.uk

Tutorial 11
Diabetes   www.diabetes.org.uk
www.diabetes-healthnet.ac.uk/leaflets/main.htm

Tutorial 15
Migraines   www.migrainetrust.org

Tutorial 16
Bereavement   Griefnet.org

Tutorial 19
Sleep apnoea   www.britishsnoring.demon.co.uk
Sleep disorders   www.familydoctor.org/handouts/212/html

Tutorial 20
Stroke rehabilitation   www.jr2.ox.ac.uk/Bandolier/band3/b3-2.html
Stroke   www.stroke.org.uk

Tutorial 22
Cystitis   www.patient.co.uk

Index